# Health in the City

# Related Titles

**Nadel & Oberlander**  TREES IN THE CITY
**Pederson**  TRANSPORTATION IN CITIES
**Catalano**  HEALTH, BEHAVIOR AND THE COMMUNITY
**Mushkin & Dunlop**  HEALTH: WHAT IS IT WORTH?
**Cappon & Zakus**  HEALTH AND THE ENVIRONMENT
**Duhl & Den Boer**  MAKING WHOLE: HEALTH FOR A NEW EPOCH

# Health in the City

## Environmental and Behavioral Influences

Malcolm S. Weinstein

### Pergamon Press
New York • Oxford • Toronto • Sydney • Frankfurt • Paris

*Pergamon Press Offices:*

W 424

**U.S.A**  Pergamon Press Inc., Maxwell House, Fairview Park, Elmsford, New York 10523, U.S.A.

**U.K.**  Pergamon Press Ltd., Headington Hill Hall, Oxford OX3 0BW, England

**CANADA**  Pergamon of Canada Ltd., 150 Consumers Road, Willowdale, Ontario M2J 1P9, Canada

**AUSTRALIA**  Pergamon Press (Aust) Pty. Ltd., P.O. Box 544, Potts Point, NSW 2011, Australia

**FRANCE**  Pergamon Press SARL, 24 rue des Ecoles, 75240 Paris, Cedex 05, France

**FEDERAL REPUBLIC OF GERMANY**  Pergamon Press GmbH, 6242 Kronberg/Taunus, Pferdstrasse 1, Federal Republic of Germany

614.7
W 424

**Library of Congress Cataloging in Publication Data**

Weinstein, Malcolm S     1942-
   Health in the city.

   (Habitat texts)
   Bibliography: p.
   Includes index.
   1.  Urban health.  2.  Medical care.  I.  Title.
II.  Series.  [DNLM:  1.  Health.  2.  Environmental
health—United States.  3.  Urban health.  WA380 W424h]
RA566.7.W44  1979     614.7′09173′2     79-13834
ISBN 0-08-023375-9

*Printed in the United States of America*

To my wife, Judy, and my sons,
Jason and Todd, whose love and
friendship do so much for my own
health in the city.

# Contents

List of Figures and Tables                                    ix

List of Health Notes                                          xi

Preface                                                       xiii

Acknowledgments                                               xvii

Chapter
  1  HEALTH IN THE CITY TODAY: DO
      CITIES MAKE US SICK?                               1

  2  HEALTH IN THE CITY YESTERDAY: PEOPLE,
      PESTS, AND POLLUTION THROUGH THE AGES             13

  3  THE PHYSICAL ENVIRONMENT: EAT, DRINK –
      BUT DON'T BREATHE THE AIR!                        25

  4  THE RESIDENTIAL AND SOCIAL ENVIRONMENT:
      DON'T FENCE ME IN!                                39

  5  BEHAVIORAL AND PSYCHOSOCIAL FACTORS:
      IS IT ALL IN MY MIND?                             47

  6  HEALTH CARE IN THE CITY: THERE'S ONLY
      ONE THING WRONG WITH HOSPITALS – TOO
      MANY SICK PEOPLE                                  61

  7  HEALTH IN THE CITY TOMORROW: A RETURN
      TO HYGEIA, THE CITY OF HEALTH                     69

Appendixes
  A: Health Statistics and Health
      Resources                                      75

  B:  Health Games                               79

Annotated Bibliography                             85

Index                                              89

About the Author                                   93

# List of Figures
# and Tables

| Figure | 1.1 | Urban Population Increases: 1800-2000 | 4 |
| | 1.2 | Average Life Expectancy from Prehistoric to Modern Times | 7 |
| | 1.3 | Life Expectancy at Birth for Selected Countries by Sex, 1972 | 8 |
| | 5.1 | The Health Belief Model (Simplified Form) | 59 |
| Table | 1.1 | Leading Causes of Death in the U.S. in 1866, 1916, and 1974 | 10 |
| | 3.1 | History of Water Treatment Processes and Water Distribution Milestones | 28 |
| | 3.2 | Decibel Levels of Common Sounds | 33 |
| | 3.3 | Life Expectancy Lost per 65 Years Due to Radiation | 34 |
| | 5.1 | Social Readjustment Rating Scale | 53 |
| | 5.2 | Model for Health Policy Analysis: Disease Evaluation | 56 |

# List of
# Health Notes

Epidemiology of Coronary Heart Disease Mortality                    9
Plague                                                            16
Cholera                                                           19
Typhoid (or Enteric) Fever                                        20
Excerpt from a Special Hearing Held by the Select
    Committee on the Health of Towns (1840)                       21
Emphysema                                                         30
Some Research Results                                             30
DDT and Death                                                     36
Housing and Health in Developing Countries                        41
Type A Behavior and Coronary Heart Disease                        49
Smoking                                                           57
Nutrition                                                         58
Health Care in Big Cities                                         62
Hospitals in the Nineteenth Century                               64
Stanford Heart Disease Prevention Program                         66
The Tao of Health                                                 67

# Preface

This book is about health in cities and shows how city life influences and reflects our physical and mental health. It influences the water we drink, the housing we live in, the treatment of our bodies and minds, and the health services we provide for ourselves.

Today's city has the potential to meet our physical needs better than ever before; modern technology has been developed to assure clean water and effective sanitation services even for large cities. Many communicable diseases such as typhoid and cholera, which resulted from hazards of our physical environment, have been dramatically controlled. At the same time, the prevalence of chronic diseases of the heart and lung, accidents, and mental disorders has risen dramatically. While the city has witnessed dramatic physical improvements over the past 100 years in relation to communicable diseases, it has a long way to go to promote the kinds of social environments and healthy lifestyles required to cut down on chronic diseases.

The modern city developed out of man's need to cope with his physical environment. Many of today's urban health problems arose during the period of accelerated urbanization brought about by the industrial revolution in the nineteenth century. Thousands of people rushed from rural areas into cities to seek their fortunes in the fields of manufacturing and commerce. These rapid influxes of people strained the resources of small towns.

City governments were forced to react to health concerns. Some of our earliest city bylaws and departments were created to deal with such issues as water quality, the burial of the dead (to protect citizens from spread of infection), and sewage treatment. Physical problems were given a great deal of early attention while the seeds of social and health problems resulting from overcrowding and poor housing were ignored. Today's health in the city reflects this early priority of physical over social needs. This book argues that health and city planning today must correct this imbalance if we wish to improve the level of health in the city tomorrow.

Why focus on the city? The answer is simple. The majority of people in Western society now live in urban settings. And as other nations shift from rural to industrial economies they, too, will become urbanized. In fact, by the year 2000 it is expected that over 70 percent of the world's population will live in cities.

Urban settings, compared with rural ones, have higher population densities (more people per area), higher educational levels, more diverse and specialized occupations, less seasonal unemployment, more varied lifestyles, and higher income levels. They also have more environmental pollution, unemployment, traffic congestion, inadequate housing, and expensive services. What do all these factors, individually and collectively, mean for our health? How do they affect personal relationships between city dwellers? Are they, for example, lonelier than their rural counterparts? This book will try to answer these and other questions related to health in the city.

## WHAT IS HEALTH?

Health is a difficult concept to define. Some define it in terms of longevity — the number of years we live. Others define health in terms of what it is not — health is not having a disease. For others, health refers to a balance of energy between the body and the mind and in the relationship between the person and the world around him.

The World Health Organization defines health as "a state of complete physical, emotional and social well-being and not merely the absence of disease and infirmity." (WHO, 1958, p. 459) Health is a result of elements in the person, the environment, and the health system itself. Personal elements might be genetic (a predisposition to a high level of "cholesterol" in the blood, a disease such as sickle cell anemia), constitutional (weight and height), or behavioral (smoking or exercise). Environmental elements include both physical and social factors outside the person's skin. Air and water pollution are part of the physical environment. Importantly, the health system itself influences health. The quality, quantity, accessibility, and cost of health services — even our beliefs about health — all contribute to our state of health.

It is a commonly believed myth that country life is healthier than city life. Statistics are quoted to show that urban death rates are higher than rural ones. It is a fact that a high mortality rate has traditionally limited the growth of cities. During the industrial revolution in the 1850s, the life expectancy of a person living in London was only 36 years, and as late as 1901-1910, the death rate for the urban counties in England and Wales, even after adjusting the samples for age differences,

---

Cholesterol: A fatty compound in the blood that is found in deposits on the walls of arteries. It is a factor in heart disease.

was 33 percent higher than the death rate for rural counties. Yet such statistics are misleading today. In the first place, urban-rural differences are found for only some diseases, and usually only for males. If city life is the culprit, why are females not equally affected? Moreover, since older people suffer more from disease and disability than younger ones, and since there are significantly more older people in cities than in rural areas, higher statistics may simply reflect this age difference. Finally, statistics may reflect the fact that the city's specialized health services act as a magnet for ill people who might otherwise remain in rural areas.

Cities are better equipped to fight certain health problems than they were 100 years ago. But to achieve similar gains against today's killers – heart disease, cancer, accidents, and suicide – we must stop abusing our physical environment, our bodies, and other people. We must alter our lifestyles and design our cities with these needs in mind.

City planning began with health concerns. The fundamental need of ancient and modern cities for clean water and sanitation requires effective planning of pipes and sewers. Health planning can be viewed as a specialized field of overall planning, where quality of life is expressed in health terms; the number of years of healthy life lived, days free from illness, and other indicators are the yardsticks against which progress is measured. The goal of both the health and city planner alike is to design services and facilities that make the best use of the resources available to achieve health in the city.

## PLAN OF THE BOOK

Seven chapters organize the text. Chapter 1 provides facts and figures about urbanization and health today and introduces basic terminology from "demography" to "epidemiology." Chapter 2 provides a historical look at these issues. Chapter 3 outlines the impact of the physical environment – polluted air and water, toxic chemicals, radiation, and other components – on health. Chapter 4, which discusses the impact on

City planners can make sure that the physical environment does not create additional sources of stress in people's lives, and more positively, that it gives them as much satisfaction as possible.

In addition to removing sources of stress wherever possible, city planners can also make sure that the physical environment will give people as much satisfaction as possible, and help them live the way they want to live.

– Herbert Gans, Planning – and City Planning – for Mental Health, 1967

health of residential and social environments, includes topics such as housing, crowding, and poverty. The critical role of behavioral and psychological factors such as stress and lifestyles (smoking, alcohol use, nutrition, fitness) on health, particularly on chronic diseases, is the subject of chapter 5. Chapter 6 shows that the cost of providing health care in the city is too high. A less expensive system of health care oriented to prevention as well as cure is needed. Finally, chapter 7 discusses the implications of the previous chapters for health in the city tomorrow. Sources of information, health games, and materials for further study are given in Appendixes A and B.

Demography: The statistical study of life events such as births, deaths, and marriages in populations.

Epidemiology: The study of disease and health patterns and their causes in populations.

# Acknowledgments

This book was written with help from a lot of people and places. My thanks to Professor Ira Nadel, editor of this Habitat Text series, who tried his best to teach me how to write English; my colleagues at the Vancouver Health Department who read and gave me valuable comments on earlier drafts and ideas for this book — particularly Dr. Roberta McQueen, Dr. Gerald Bonham, and Guy Costanzo; and all the other health and urban studies people with whom I talked during its writing. And special thanks to Rey Castro and Brenda Seehuber who managed somehow to decipher my scrawls and translate them into type.

My sincere thanks, too, to the institutions and organizations that provided consultation and/or materials in the writing of this book: the Vancouver Health Department, Vancouver City Archives, Vancouver Public Library, Gibson Medical Library at the University of British Columbia, and the Department of National Health and Welfare of the Government of Canada (for permission to use material from Operation Lifestyle).

# 1 Health in the City Today: Do Cities Make Us Sick?

Many people believe that health in the city today is worse than it was 100 years ago. This book examines the evidence for this belief and comes to a somewhat surprising conclusion – people who live in cities are not only healthier than they were 100 years ago, in many respects their health is superior to that of people who live in the country. Yet this hard-won improvement in health could be lost if we do not make radical changes both in our expensive health care systems and in our own personal health practices.

It is a fact that the death rate in urban areas, particularly for men, is still higher than in rural areas. But this difference is decreasing. And whether city or rural death rates are worse depends upon the cause of death being considered. If you are between 15 and 24 years of age, you are more likely to die from a motor vehicle accident than from anything else. The chances are even higher if you live in a rural area. For other causes of death, such as chronic diseases of the circulatory system (high blood pressure), respiratory system (asthma or diseases of the lung), or digestive system (ulcers, cirrhosis of the liver), the evidence is mixed, although rates are slightly higher in cities. Today's city dweller is more likely to die from a chronic disease like heart disease than from an infectious disease like tuberculosis. Formerly, a newborn baby had a poor chance for survival in the city, but this situation has changed. Since the 1930s and 1940s, as a result of improved hospital care in cities, infant survival rates in most Western,

What glorious sunsets have their birth
In Cities fouled by smoke!
This tree – whose roots are in a drain –
Becomes the greenest oak.

-W.H. Davies, "Love's Rivals," 1935

1

industrialized nations such as the U.S., Canada, and Sweden have surpassed rural rates.

The question of whether people in cities are healthier than they used to be depends on how we define cities and measure health. This chapter explores these two basic concepts which are grouped under the headings urbanization and health. It also presents some facts and figures about city populations and health problems today.

## THE GROWTH OF CITIES AND URBANIZATION

Cities first appeared about 5,500 years ago. They were small settlements within an overwhelmingly rural society. Written records show that the world's first major cities took shape around 3500 B.C. in the valleys of the Tigris and Euphrates rivers. The early cities shared a similar technological base consisting of wheat and barley as cereal crops, bronze as the metal, and animals as energy sources. Cities became the centers for the ruling elite – the religious, political, military, and commercial leaders – as well as the focal point for the laborers, craftsmen, and professionals who served the ruling class.

Urbanization – the gradual shift of scattered rural populations to settlements of several thousand people – is a fairly recent development in our social evolution. While the definition of "urban" varies somewhat from country to country, a population figure of about 20,000 located in a single area is often used. The leading demographer, Kingsley Davis, notes that urbanization has taken place at a phenomenal rate. In 1965, he wrote:

> Before 1850 no society on earth could be described as predominantly urbanized, and by 1900 only one – Great Britain – could be so regarded. Today, only 65 years later, all industrial nations are highly urbanized, and in the world as a whole the process of urbanization is accelerating rapidly.

The industrial revolution of the mid-nineteenth century dramatically reversed the distribution of population between village and city. Two factors set the stage for this shift. First, the productivity of the medieval agricultural system was inadequate. Not enough production was realized per person. Second, the medieval social system of feudal lords and their serfs began to break down. Not enough production of food meant that communities had to trade and to manufacture goods to trade.  People moved from villages to towns in order to produce specialized goods. With craftsmen living in towns, merchants could more easily control their activities and costs of production. This early connection between industry and commerce set the stage for the eventual breakthroughs in urbanization during the industrial revolution by uniting productivity with consumption.

Population shifts and rates of growths after industrialization are striking. In sixteenth-century Europe, cities of 100,000 people made up only about 1.6 percent of the population. This proportion was 20 percent by 1841 and 40 percent by 1900. In 1800 only about 6 percent of the U.S. population lived in cities; today that figure is more than 70 percent. In 1850, only four cities in the world had a population of 1 million or more. Forecasts call for 275 cities of 1 million or more people by the year 2000.

The later a country becomes industrialized, the faster the process of urbanization takes place. Changes from a situation in which only 10 percent of the population lived in cities of 100,000 or more to one in which over 30 percent did so took 79 years in England and Wales, 66 years in the United States and Canada, 48 years in Germany, 36 years in Japan, and only 26 years in Australia.

Demographers have compiled data on world and local urbanization patterns over the 20-year period, 1950-1970. According to their projections, there will be a dramatic reversal from a 60 percent rate of rural dwellers to about a 61.5 percent rate of urban dwellers by the year 2000. Of the world's 7 billion people, about 4.2 billion will be "urbanites."

Urbanization and the growth of cities are often incorrectly seen as a single process. They are not. Urbanization refers to the shift from rural to urban patterns of settlement; city growth refers to population increases of established cities and their suburbs. Even after urbanization ceases, cities will continue to grow as long as births outnumber deaths. For example, between 1945 and 1961 the population of New Zealand that was classified as urban increased only slightly from 61.3 percent to 63.6 percent while the population of New Zealand's cities increased by 50 percent.

Figure 1.1 shows how world urbanization patterns have shifted since 1800. Urbanization rates today are highest in the developing countries, especially in Africa. The health changes we will discuss in this book may give us some clues about future urban health patterns in developing countries.

A city has little effect on health by itself. Urbanization influences health through such things as increased population density, more variety in terms of occupation (fewer agricultural workers), a higher general level of education, better health services, and different kinds of personal relationships and lifestyles.

## THE CONCEPT OF HEALTH

Health is a concept we all use, as well as a subject of study, but it still remains difficult to define. The World Health Organization in 1958 provided this definition: "Health is a state of complete physical, emotional, and social well-being and not merely the absence of disease or infirmity." (WHO, 1958)

In other words health is not just the absence of disease; it includes the idea of positive health or "well-being." Health has to do with balance and harmony. The ancient Greeks talked about internal balance among four basic elements of life — earth, air, water, and fire:

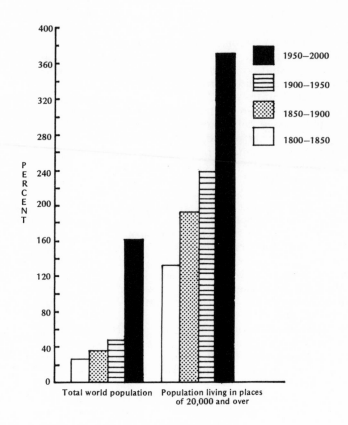

Fig. 1.1. Urban Population Increases: 1800-2000
The differences in the size of increases between the sets of
bars dramatically show how population has become concen-
trated in urban areas.

There are four natures out of which the body is compacted, earth and fire and water and air, and the unnatural excess or defect of these, or the change of any of them from its own natural place into another, or — since there are more kinds than one of fire and of the other elements — the assumption by any of these of a wrong kind, or any similar irregularity, produces disorders and diseases. . . .

— Plato, Timaeus, ca. 400 B.C.

Modern writers who talk in terms of biochemical and electrical energy balances have the same basic idea in mind as did Plato. Rene Dubos, an important modern thinker in the field of health, believes health involves successful adaptation to a changing environment. The healthy person or species is the one that has the capacity to learn and adapt to changing conditions. Failure to adapt means death. In summary, health is a positive state involving a balance of internal and external forces in adaptation to a changing environment. Health in the city reflects man's capacity to adapt to urban change.

## EPIDEMIOLOGY AND BASIC INDICATORS OF HEALTH

Epidemiology is the science that studies patterns of health and disease in human populations — how often, where, and in what kinds of people health and disease are located. Originally epidemiology was concerned with epidemics — outbreaks of disease in greater numbers than usual. Today epidemiology is a foundation science for preventive medicine and health planning. Many programs are curing and even preventing health problems — cancer, cholera, dental disease, heart disease — have benefited from the facts, figures, and hunches of epidemiologists. Since our concern is with patterns of disease and health in relation to urban settings, the point of view in this book can be called epidemiological.

Epidemiologists have developed ways to measure our health status. Unfortunately, most health status measures reflect only the presence or absence of disease rather than a positive state of health. Indicators of health status include mortality and morbidity rates, the "incidence" and "prevalence" of disease.

---

The English word "health" comes from the Old English, "hal" or "hael-th." The word "heal" means to make whole.

Epidemiology: The study of health and disease patterns in human populations.

Incidence: The number of new cases occurring during a given period of time in a population.

## Mortality Rates

The most commonly used indicator of health of a population is called the "crude mortality rate" – the number of people in a given population who die within a given period of time. This is called a "crude" rate because it lumps much information (rather crudely) into a single statistic. For example, the crude mortality rate does not tell us whether death rates differ for age groups, sex, geographic locations, or ethnic groups. Crude death rates could be analyzed to determine whether in a particular city men die from coronary heart diseases more often than women. Analysis by sex would be useful in the development of a program to prevent heart disease. A different educational approach to men and women might be used if men were found to have a greater "risk" of dying from this particular disease than women. There is no need to analyze a crude rate unless more details are needed for some other purposes such as planning health programs.

Another way to look at the crude mortality rate is by examining "life expectancy" – the average number of years a person of a certain age can expect to live. This kind of information is used by actuaries in constructing life insurance tables and determining the costs of pre-miums. Life expectancy data can be broken down into finer and finer detail depending upon the type of analysis required.

Figure 1.2 shows how life expectancy has changed from prehistoric to modern times. We now expect to live more than twice as long as our Neanderthal ancestors. Why? One reason is our extended life span due to a dramatic decrease in the rate of infant mortality. If more babies live, the average life span increases whether or not people actually live longer.

In the 40-year period from 1931 to 1971 in Canada, life expectancy for a newborn male increased from 60.0 to 69.3 years. Life expectancy for females has increased even more, from 62.1 years in 1931 – about 3.5 percent longer than for males – to 76.4 years in 1971 – 10.2 percent longer than for males.

Figure 1.3 compares life expectancy for each sex in ten major industrial nations. Although we hear stories from time to time of people in remote, underdeveloped villages living 100 years or more, the highest life expectancy today is found in an advanced country, Sweden. Life expectancy is generally not related to urbanization, to the number of physicians available, or to any other single measure, though it does reflect the care given to mothers and newborns.

―――

Prevalence: The total number of cases – old and new – existing in a given period of time in a population.

Crude Mortality Rate: The number of people in a given population who die within a given period of time.

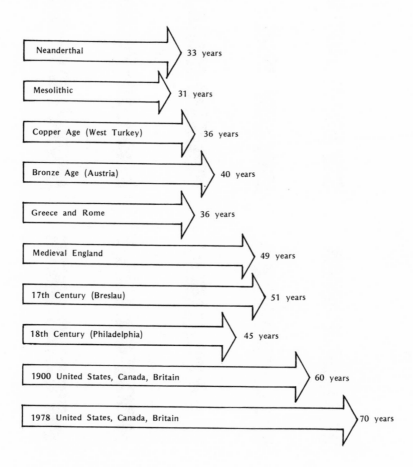

Fig. 1.2. Average Life Expectancy from Prehistoric to Modern Times

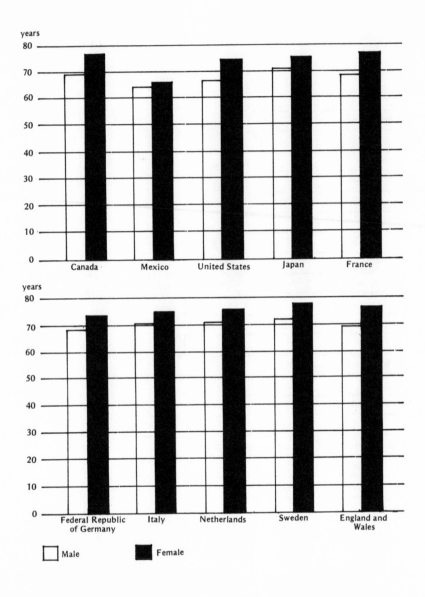

Fig. 1.3. Life Expectancy at Birth for Selected Countries by Sex, 1972
Comment: Most countries show similar life expectancies, with Sweden at the top. Women clearly expect to live longer than men.

Crude mortality rates are often further analyzed as to the major cause of death. Table 1.1 compares the ten leading causes of death in the United States for the years 1866, 1916, and 1974. Causes of death also differ according to age and sex. In the U.S. males and females in the 15-24 year age group are more likely to die from motor vehicle accidents than from anything else. In the middle years heart disease has its greatest impact. For middle-aged females, cancer is a greater risk than heart disease. The statistics for suicide are higher during early and middle adulthood, particularly for males.

Another useful mortality rate is the "infant mortality rate." This rate refers to the number of live born newborns and infants who die within their first year of life. It can be further subdivided, if necessary, for rates of deaths within the first week or month of life. Over 40 percent of infant deaths in the U.S. occur in the first day of life, 25 percent in the first week (excluding first day), and 5 percent in the first month (excluding first week). Only 6 percent of infant deaths occur in the second half of the first year. Infant mortality figures for different countries show Sweden, the Netherlands, Finland, and Norway in the lead with less than 15 infant deaths per 1,000 live births. With all their wealth and medical expertise, countries like Canada and the U.S. place no better than thirteenth and fourteenth, respectively, in these rankings.

The number of infant deaths is an end product of a great many contributing factors such as the mother's general nutritional, physical, and emotional health, the quality and availability of health and obstetrical services, and so on. Since many of these contributing factors differ in urban and rural settings, urban-rural differences in mortality rates may be expected.

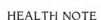

### HEALTH NOTE

#### Epidemiology Of Coronary Heart Disease Mortality

Epidemiologists Drs. Herman Tyroler and John Cassel at the University of North Carolina in 1964 studied differences in coronary heart disease mortality in two groups. The first group was made up of middle-aged American males of British ancestry. These men had been raised in rural settings which became urbanized during their lifetimes. These men, therefore, experienced urbanization, but did not change their place of residence. A second group was made up of men raised in exclusively urban conditions all their lives. A ten-year follow-up showed that the urban group had a greater increase in coronary heart disease mortality than did the gradually urbanized group.

Table 1.1. Leading Causes of Death in the U.S. in 1866, 1916, And 1974

| | 1866 | | 1916 | | 1974 |
|---|---|---|---|---|---|
| 1. | Diarrheal diseases | 1. | Heart disease | 1. | Heart disease |
| 2. | Diarrheal diseases under 5 | 2. | Pneumonia | 2. | Cancer |
| 3. | All diseases of the nervous system | 3. | Pulmonary tuberculosis | 3. | Cerebrovascular disease |
| 4. | Phthisis (pulmonary tuberculosis) | 4. | Bright's disease and nephritis | 4. | Accidents |
| 5. | Pneumonia | 5. | Violence | 5. | Influenza and pneumonia |
| 6. | Accidents, homicides, suicides | 6. | Cancer | 6. | Certain diseases of early infancy |
| 7. | Scarlet fever | 7. | Diarrheal diseases under 5 | 7. | Diabetes mellitus |
| 8. | Heart disease | 8. | Other tuberculosis diseases | 8. | General arteriosclerosis |
| 9. | Bronchitis | 9. | Diphtheria and croup | 9. | Cirrhosis of the liver |
| 10. | Typhoid fever | 10. | Bronchitis | 10. | Bronchitis, emphysema, and asthma |

Note the dramatic shift of heart disease, a chronic disease, from 8th to 1st place, and the recent rise for cancer. Tuberculosis, a lethal infectious disease 100 years ago, no longer appears in the top 10.

## Morbidity Rates

Not all diseases are fatal. "Morbidity rates" give a rough indication of the day-to-day health of a population by measuring such things as days lost from school, absenteeism from work, the number of days spent by patients in hospitals for various illnesses, and visits to physicians. Some countries and regions conduct periodic morbidity and health surveys for purposes of health planning. The U.S. established a National Health Survey in 1956 and similar surveys have taken place in England, Wales, and Denmark.

Special surveys for specific diseases such as cancer are also undertaken from time to time. While mortality rates are generally higher for men than women, these national surveys show that women have higher morbidity rates. This sex difference is found consistently in both rural and urban settings. In fact, urban female mortality and morbidity rates are climbing. These changes in statistics for women may reflect the fact that more and more women are being exposed to the same economic and occupational pressures traditionally hazardous to men.

## Interpreting Urban-Rural Differences

It is difficult to interpret data on city and country differences in health because factors other than urbanization may be causing the differences. For example, urban-rural differences may result from the fact that people who live in cities are older on the average than their rural counterparts. So death rates may be higher in cities simply because more older people die. Statistics may also be misleading because of the method by which they are reported. Many people from rural areas die in hospitals in urban areas; if deaths are recorded according to place of death rather than place of residence, this artificially inflates city rates. Also, distinctions between "rural" and "urban" areas are never pure. Urban and rural areas are in fact mixtures of different concentrations of populations — towns, suburbs, cities. People move among these settings throughout their lifetimes. Thus, the urban-rural distinction should be recognized for what it is — a simplified way of looking at the question of how health and density of population are related.

## SUMMING UP

As a result of gains made in man's battle against infectious disease, health in the city today is better than it was 100 years ago. Yet epidemiological studies show that life in cities is associated with in-

---

Morbidity Rates: The proportion of people in a given population who become ill during a given period of time.

creasing incidence and prevalence rates of chronic health problems, heart disease, and suicide.

Yesterday's advances must be maintained; however, if similar gains are to be made against chronic disease, then health planners, city planners, health professionals, and citizens must work together more closely than ever before to prevent illness and promote well-being.

Chapter 2 traces the historical roots of our current urban health problems. It also describes some pioneering efforts to achieve health reform.

———

The health of the people is really the foundation upon which all their happiness and all their powers as a State depend.
— Prime Minister Disraeli of England, 1877

# 2 Health in the City Yesterday: People, Pests, and Pollution through the Ages

Today's urban health problems — communicable diseases, pollution, chronic disease — can be examined from three points of view: environmental, bacterial, and ecological. Each point of view represents a stage in the history of health in the city.

The first stage was environmental sanitation, originating in ancient Greece and Rome. The belief that health problems were the result of airborne particles, or "miasma" led the Greeks and Romans to develop methods to improve water supplies and to treat waste and sewage. They also recognized behavioral influences on health, such as diet and physical fitness, but gave these factors less attention than environmental issues.

The second stage was bacterial. It was centered in Europe, particularly England. The invention of the microscope and an accelerating pace of scientific experimentation in the eighteenth and nineteenth centuries led to the exciting discovery that microorganisms such as "bacteria" could cause diseases and that "inoculation" could prevent them. In this phase, environmental concerns with water and waste were overshadowed, though people were beginning to recognize the potential health hazards of polluted air from new industrial developments.

The first two stages focused on the prevention of dreaded communicable diseases, particularly typhoid, cholera, and plague. A third stage, which is now emerging, is the ecological stage. Here, earlier concerns with both environmental and behavioral factors are considered together. The focus of the health field is on chronic diseases such as

———

Bacteria: One-celled organisms, some of which cause disease.

Inoculation: An injection of a serum or antibody to prevent or cure a disease.

heart disease, cancer, and mental disorders, as well as accidents, particularly those involving motor vehicles. Increased awareness of ecological issues in the 1960s – scarce national resources, the inter-dependence of people and the planet, air and water pollution – has led to a greater awareness of man's need to work in partnership with nature.

The theme of health as balance and harmony, central to the writings of the ancient Greeks and Eastern cultures, is reemerging. Concerns with better personal health habits are being voiced by individuals and even governments. A Canadian government document entitled "A New Perspective on the Health of Canadians" (1974) states that self-imposed risks such as smoking, poor nutrition, lack of fitness, and excessive stress and alcohol consumption are major contributors to heart disease, cancer, cirrhosis of the liver, and motor vehicle accidents. The hordes of early morning joggers present throughout North America illustrate a reaction against those harmful habits.

Just as the environmental sanitation stage was based upon the miasma theory and the bacterial stage on the germ theories of microbiology, the ecological stage draws upon the behavioral and social sciences for its concepts and methods. The goal of the ecological stage is the ancient ideal of a healthy mind in a healthy body in a healthful environment.

## HEALTH PRACTICES IN ANCIENT CIVILIZATIONS

The history of urban health goes back thousands of years. Information on environmental concerns such as impurities of water, and personal health problems such as communicable diseases exists in the Bible. Old Testament writings in Leviticus and in Numbers discuss such communi-cable diseases as "leprosy" and provide instructions for the preparation of nutritious foods and household disinfectants.

Archeologists have unearthed some of the earliest examples of urban health practices. Ruins in the Indus valley and the Punjab in India dating back to 4000 B.C. suggest the inhabitants were well advanced in sanitary engineering. They also indicate that building codes were in effect. The early Egyptians (2000 B.C.) and Incas built housing that contained bathroom facilities and elaborate sewage systems.    The Minoans on the Greek island of Crete built the first latrine and flush toilet in about 1000 B.C.

Antibodies: Proteins in the blood formed in reaction to foreign proteins. They neutralize foreign proteins and produce immunity from them.

Leprosy: A chronic bacterial disease marked by slow-growing swellings with deformity and loss of feeling in the affected parts.

The ancient Greeks and Romans made the greatest contributions to urban health. The Greeks viewed health as a harmonious balance between the mind and body. Their emphasis on personal health, physical fitness, and strength (primarily for their ruling classes) helped those who survived birth to achieve high levels of health. Unfortunately, so few newborns survived that it was customary for the Greeks to wait a week before naming a newborn child.

The Greeks were also concerned with environmental influences on health. Hipprocrates, the "father" of medicine, wrote in 400 B.C. in his famous work On Airs, Waters, and Places:

> Whoever wishes to investigate medicine properly, should proceed thus: in the first place to consider the seasons of the year, and what effects each of them produces, for they are not at all alike, but differ much from themselves in regard to their changes. . . . We must also consider the qualities of the waters. . . whether they be marshy and soft, or hard. . . .

Before the modern science of bacteriology developed, physicians used the "miasmatic" (contaminating atmosphere) theory of the Greeks to explain the cause of diseases and to suggest possible treatments. As we shall see in later chapters, the miasmatic theory has been reappearing in recent years as polluted city environments are identified as causing certain diseases.

The ancient Romans made tremendous contributions to urban health in the fields of community sanitation, occupational health, and health service facilities. They built at least 14 sophisticated aqueducts to transport water to Rome from mountains and, in 600 B.C., developed a sewage system, services for garbage removal and street cleaning, and laws for the regulation of public bars and prostitution. They also devised crude respirators to protect workers from dust, and built the first hospitals called "leprosariums" for the isolation of sufferers from leprosy.

Other early cultures in China, India, and in the Arab world also developed public health measures. Inoculation against smallpox, reintroduced into modern health practice only recently, was practiced in India and China in pre-Christian times. Early Arab civilizations even had health departments with staffs of health inspectors to ensure that their citizens enjoyed clean food.

In spite of these examples of early enlightenment, health problems in ancient times were serious. As cities developed, the problems increased. In Rome, crowding and squalor provided a breeding ground for disease. Most health benefits were accessible only to the ruling elite. Epidemic diseases such as malaria went unchecked. The population of the world advanced from about 275 million to only 450 million during the 500 years from A.D. 1000 to A.D. 1500. In contrast, current population trends indicate we will see the world's population double by the year 2000.

Early urban dwellers ignored problems of maternal and child health, infant mortality, and occupational hazards. In A.D. 157, in his text De

Sanitate Tuenda, the Roman physician Galen wrote:

> The life of men is involved in the business of their occupation and it is inevitable that they should be harmed by what they do... and it is impossible to change it.

## THE MIDDLE AGES AND THE RENAISSANCE

Health measures developed by earlier cultures declined in the Middle Ages (A.D. 500-1500). Town councils, drawn from among the wealthier citizens, had to develop methods for dealing efficiently with health problems of many more people, including those whose health habits were less sophisticated than theirs. Congestion and exposure to harmful bacteria set the stage for disease and death.

Some medieval monasteries had proper water supplies and heating and ventilation facilities but most places did not. Most medieval cities had difficulty providing their citizens with a sufficient supply of nonpolluted water. In England, laws were enacted against acts of public mischief such as pollution of water and other threats to public health. In 1271, in Douai, France, a law was passed which forbade tanners to wash animal skins on the banks of the streams; early in the fifteenth century, several German cities outlawed the construction of hogpens facing the street. Paris, in 1185, paved its city streets in order to facilitate their cleaning; London passed ordinances in 1309 to deal with sewage and disposal; Milan in the 1300s passed statutes regulating cesspools and sewers. Unfortunately, most of these laws were not strictly enforced.

Plagues were particularly devastating during the Middle Ages. The worst of these was the Black Death or bubonic plague which spread over Europe from 1348 to 1350. Approximately one out of every four people died as a result of this epidemic; England's population dropped by one-third from 3.8 to 2.1 million persons. In an effort to halt the spread of

### HEALTH NOTE

#### Plague

Plague is an infectious disease which attacks rats. Humans become infected from a bite by a flea from an infected rat. A few days after the bite the patient has a fever and headache. He becomes drowsy and staggers about as if drunk. In bubonic plague painful swelling called buboes form in the groin or under the arms. In another form of disease, pneumonic plague, the lungs become inflamed and the patient has difficulty in breathing.

the plague, the practice of quarantining incoming ships was adopted. While there has never again been a large-scale outbreak of this devastating plague, cases of bubonic and other plagues still occur (see Health Note).

A rebirth of learning took place in Italy and other European countries during the Renaissance period (from about the fourteenth to the seventeenth century). Many ancient Greek and Roman medical treatises which had been preserved by monks during the Middle Ages were discovered and progress was made in the organization of medical care. A number of Italian city-states developed procedures for community sanitation. On the whole, though, the Renaissance was not a period for great leaps forward in urban health. It was, however, a time for making exciting scientific discoveries about human anatomy and physiology. The Italian physician, Vesalius, took advantage of the Church's relaxation of the prohibition against dissection of cadavers and produced a major work on human anatomy. In England, Sir William Harvey produced his classic text on the circulation of blood. These and other discoveries laid the foundation for progress in public and urban health during the sanitary movement of the mid-nineteenth century.

## THE SANITARY MOVEMENT OF THE 1850s

The mid-1800s marked the beginning of modern urban health. Increased urbanization sharpened the contrasts between city and country life.

Probably true was the stereotype of the country dweller, in contrast to the urban dweller, having more fresh air, cleaner water (usually from his own well), private sanitary facilities with appropriate sewage treatment, and a better diet of fresh vegetables, fruit, and milk. The towns were characterized by dirt and smell, particularly smells of horse dung and waste from the tanneries and slaughter houses. A visitor to Manchester, England, described this scene in 1832:

> I have seen the lowest quarters of Marseilles, Antwerp and Paris: they come nowhere near this. Squat houses, wretched streets of brick under red roofs crossing each other in all directions and leading dismally down to the river,. . .narrow alleys, and dusty yards, were foul with the smell of rotting old clothes and decorated with rags and linen hung out to dry. . . .The houses are generally of a single story, low, dilapidated, kennels to sleep and die in. . . .The impression is not one of debauchery, but of abject, miserable poverty. One is sickened and wounded by this deplorable procession. . . .Here is a festering sore, the real sore on the body of English society.
>
> – From an account by Hyppolyte Taine (1828-93) as reported in Longmate, 1970.

## Sanitation

It was common practice in the Middle Ages to keep all domestic rubbish, including human excrement, in the house until residents could no longer stand it, and then throw it into a central space. Doctors attending the sick or delivering a new baby had to make frequent trips outside the house to breathe relatively fresher air. The problem was aggravated, as one might imagine, in hot weather!

In most towns, clean water was an even scarcer commodity than fresh air. In the 1830s only wealthy families had water piped directly into their homes, and then only for a few hours daily. Running water from a pump was cause for great excitement in a district; maids and common people would line up for their share of the precious liquid. Water obtained in this manner was generally brought indoors and stored in open buckets. It was often covered by a kind of black "scum." Water selling was a profitable business at a half-penny a bucket.

While there were some public pumps, they were very rare. St. Pancras, a district in central London with 170,000 inhabitants, had only 13 pumps in 1830. Where there was no water supply, people dipped their buckets into the Thames River. Unfortunately, the water was contaminated by waste from sewers and from chemicals fed directly into it from nearby factories. In view of the scarcity of good quality drinking water, it is not surprising that beer was the everyday drink. It was cheaper than clean water at two pence a pint.

Diets, except for the very poor, included bread, potatoes, meat, fish, and cheese. But people did not understand basic nutrition and the need for unadulterated (pure) foods. Grocers used to add foreign substances to foods to increase their weight (and their profit!). People were advised to examine their tea with magnets in order to test for the presence of iron filings. "Grocer's itch," a prevalent health problem, was caused by the dirt and sand mites that were added by grocers to their sugar supplies. A government study of beer between 1844 and 1856 found that 142 of 215 samples tested contained impurities.

The greatest problem of all was the problem of sanitation. A toilet was a luxury; only the very wealthy had their own facilities and, even if they did, the waste from these facilities was more likely than not to run into cesspits which were likely to overflow. One outdoor privy was shared by several families in poorer districts; rarely was it emptied or cleaned. Chamber pots were commonly used with their contents emptied out of windows onto the street or dumped in fields. Streets were often blocked to traffic by piles of human excrement. As late as 1850 there were still 250,000 cesspools in London; Birmingham spent a considerable sum of money each year on emptying privies; in Manchester fewer than 1 house in 20 had a toilet. The great irony of this situation was that the British continued to look down upon "filthy foreigners!"

### Conditions Of Work

Industrialization produced major physical and mental health problems for urban workers, particularly children. Long, unbroken hours of work in humid, poorly ventilated and dusty conditions impaired health. In certain trades a whole family might work in a single room with inadequate ventilation. Diseases flourished and their spread was aided under these conditions. Outbreaks of "fevers" were common; as a result of dangerous and unfenced machinery, maiming and mutilation were routine events. Young children were a regular part of the work force from an early age. Their suffering was particularly disgusting and inhumane.

Decreased life expectancy reflected the poor sanitary and working conditions. In the mid-nineteenth century, life expectancy was less than 25 years in Britain's industrial areas but 40 years in the country as a whole. Not only were the people affected directly; the indirect effects of poor working and living conditions on the health of future generations were enormous. Malnutrition, infant diseases, poor dental health, and other health hazards early in life set a pattern for ill health and shortened life-spans. In turn, these early patterns were passed on to the succeeding generations.

### HEALTH NOTE

#### Cholera

Cholera was unknown before 1817, except for occasional outbreaks in India, despite the fact that most people in the world probably drank polluted water. Nobody knows why it began to spread across the world in that year. The epidemics in Britain were in 1831-2, 1853-4, and 1866.

Since then it has retreated toward its original home, India. Twenty three countries from Persia to Indonesia had cases of cholera from 1961 to 1965. There were a total of 14,000 deaths from the disease in 1965, most of which were in India, Pakistan, and Burma.

Epidemics of cholera have never occurred in a place with a good water supply.

Epidemic: An outbreak of disease in more people than is considered normal for the particular circumstances.

## The Cholera Epidemics

The major urban diseases during industrialization were smallpox, tuber-culosis, and cholera, usually in the form of epidemics. Yet cholera, the greatest single killer, was also the greatest single force for reform.

The first outbreak of Asiatic cholera in England took place in 1831-32. It took 50,000 lives. The next epidemic was in 1848 – another 50,000 deaths resulted. Between 1848 and 1854 cholera killed 250,000 people (see Health Note). A third epidemic in 1854 caused 20,000 deaths and in 1866, 14,000. Total? Almost 400,000 victims within slightly more than 30 years.

The biggest contribution to solving the mystery of cholera was made by Dr. John Snow, a London physician, who did more than any other single person in gathering evidence to prove a connection between the quality of local water supplies and cholera. In 1849 he published On the Mode of Communication of Cholera in which he put forth his theories comparing the incidence of cholera cases in different parts of the city. Snow found an apparent link between new cases of cholera and a certain water pump in Broad Street. Snow's careful research helped make the Broad Street pump a symbol of the science of epidemiology which his work helped to launch.

Typhoid epidemics caused 20,000 deaths annually and reinforced the outcry for health reforms. A related disease, typhus, also claimed about 4,000 lives, while in 1848 scarlet fever accounted for 20,000 deaths. Smallpox was endemic to urban areas; during the nineteenth century it caused 6,000 deaths each year. During the scarlet fever epidemic of the late 1830s, 31,000 died; in the 1871-73 epidemic, 44,000 died (see Health Note).

But epidemics were important catalysts in stimulating procras-tinating bureaucrats to act. In fact, a number of urban health develop-ments originating in Britain in the mid-1800s provide the foundation of today's urban health structure. The first, in 1837, was the appointment of William Farr as compiler of abstracts in Britain's Registrar General's Office. His job was to collect and analyze records of births, marriages,

⌒

## HEALTH NOTE

### Typhoid (or Enteric) Fever

The germs of typhoid fever are excreted by people who are suffering from the disease. "Carriers" are those who excrete the germs but show no signs of the illness. A long-lasting fever and diarrhea are typical symptoms. Ulcers may de-velop in the intestine. Until 1850 this disease was confused with other fevers, so there are no records of the number of cases before then. A typhoid vaccine was first produced in 1897 and millions of people are now protected by inocu-lation.

and deaths. His work was assisted by church records which had been used by John Graunt as early as 1677 to compile weekly death lists called "Bills of Mortality." Farr was the first person to compile vital statistics on a national level. Without such statistics, it had been impossible to get an objective picture of changing national health and social conditions. Now these statistics provided a baseline against which health changes could be compared from year to year. For the first time, it was possible to estimate the extent of disease and identify the gaps in health services.

Farr was a social reformer as well as a "biostatistician." To each rather dry statistical report during his 40-year tenure as compiler of abstracts, he attached long essays, comments, and suggestions for social change. Many of these suggestions were eventually adopted into legislation.

The second step forward in the fight against cholera and poor urban health conditions was taken as a result of increasing social concerns. In 1834 Edwin Chadwick was instrumental in getting the British Parliament to enact a new Poor Law. In 1838-39, during their investigations of London's worst slums, Chadwick, together with such colleagues as T. Southwood Smith, author of Philosophy of Health (1835-37), produced strong evidence that sickness and poverty were interrelated. Chadwick's motivation for reform was economic, not humanitarian. Sickness was expensive. Hospitals and clinics had to be built and operated to care for the sick. He argued that it would be good economics to clean up slums and reduce urban sickness, and thereby cut the costs of expensive hospital care.

In 1840, the British Parliament appointed a select committee:

> . . .to inquire into the circumstances affecting the Health of the Inhabitants of Large Towns and Populous Districts, with a View to Improved Sanatory (sic) Regulations for their Benefit, and who were empowered to Report their Observations, together with the Minutes of Evidence taken before them to the House.

> – Health of Towns Report, 1840

Although he was not a member of the commission, Chadwick drafted almost the entire report known as the Health of Towns report (see Health Note). The opening paragraph states:

> Your Committee have inquired carefully into the matters submitted to them, and find that sanatory (sic) regulations in many of the principal towns of the realm are most imperfect and neglected, and that hence result great evils, suffering, and expense, to large bodies of the community.

Biostatistics: The study of numerical information associated with biological and health problems.

As a result of the Health of Towns report, in 1847 the town of Liverpool appointed a doctor to be responsible for the health of the community – England's first medical officer of health. A Central Board of Health and local health boards were formed in 1848 as a result of the first Public Health Act. A board was mandatory only in towns where the death rate exceeded 22 per 1,000 or where one-tenth of tax payers petitioned for its creation.

Chadwick's leadership, which made such an impact on the establishment of boards of health, proved to be their undoing as well. The Central Board of Health was an aggressive force for change, perhaps too aggressive. The London Times in 1832 wrote, "We prefer to take our chance of cholera and the rest than be bullied into health." Many members of Parliament agreed. In 1854 Liverpool's Central Board was dissolved and Chadwick was fired.

## HEALTH NOTE

Excerpt From A Special Hearing Held By The
Select Committee On The Health Of Towns (1840)

George Alfred Walker, Esq. called in; and further examined. (4 June 1840)

3460. Mr. Mackinnon. You are a medical man? – I am.

3461. You have written a book on the subject of the burial of the dead in large towns, have you not? – I have.

3462. You have turned your attention a good deal to that subject? – I have.

3463. In the book you have published, you have mentioned the evils arising from the want of ventilation in places such as cul-de-sacs? – I have.

3464. Have the goodness to state to the Committee generally your observations upon that subject. – . . .the place in which they lived is one of the worst in the neighbourhood, being a cul-de-sac called Wellington Court, leading out of Drurylane on the northeastern side, approached by a long and narrow passage, most disgustingly dirty, without drainage, and inhabited by characters of the poorest description; the houses appear as though they were never cleaned or whitewashed, and the abominations called filthy are here in abundance.

However, the reforms the commission recommended were not to die. The establishment of local control over sanitary conditions was made official by the Sanitary Act of 1866 and the Public Health Act of 1875. Today, every major urban center has a health officer and a board of health to monitor health in the city.

In the United States a similar pattern of epidemics and social reform took place. Great smallpox epidemics in the seventeenth and eighteenth centuries, yellow fever epidemics in New York during the American Revolution, and outbreaks of cholera in the nineteenth century led to the creation of rigid public health measures. The first city health board was created in Baltimore in 1798; Charleston, S.C. (1815) and Philadelphia (1818) soon followed.

In 1850 the Sanitary Commission of Massachusetts led by Lemuel Shattuck (the U.S. equivalent of Edwin Chadwick) published a major report. This report led to Massachusetts creating the first state board of health in 1869. A similar report in New York State by Stephen Smith in 1865 led to the creation of their state board. By 1919 all the states had their own health departments.

By the turn of the century, boards of health had been joined by a variety of other health services and agencies in their efforts to protect and promote health in the city. Hospitals, clinics, and a variety of health workers combined their efforts as the field of public health grew in size and scope.

Despite recent improvements in health care through the use of specially trained paramedical staff, expanded work functions for nurses, organ transplants, microsurgery, computer diagnosis, and a whole range of specialized technology and hardware, the health of cities remains a critical concern. A current trend is a shift from large-scale hospital-based services to more health services based in the community. Many patients who previously occupied expensive, acute-care hospital beds at a cost of over $200 per day are now receiving effective services in their homes at lower cost from specially trained homecare workers.

We are also gradually rediscovering, as the Health of Towns report indicated over 100 years ago, ways to prevent disease by improving our physical and social environments. Health maintenance organizations, better methods for collecting and using health statistics for planning health services, and national health insurance schemes can trace their origins to the pioneering efforts reviewed in this chapter. Edwin Chadwick argued that it made good economic sense to reduce sickness. Today's soaring health care costs prove Chadwick's view was right.

## SUMMING UP

Health in cities has progressed through three stages of development: bacterial, environmental sanitation, and ecological. Each stage originated in ancient times and remains with us today. Environmental sanitation issues provided the foundation for urban health awareness. Control of dreaded epidemics of infectious diseases like cholera and typhoid provided motivation for reform. Social and health reforms in the 1850s laid the groundwork for legislation and the creation of local boards of health all over the world. Early concerns with poor social conditions and health were eventually overshadowed by emphasis on bacterial causes of disease. However, as we will see in subsequent chapters, an ecological view of health is now emerging, a view which takes into account environmental, bacterial, and social factors.

# 3 The Physical Environment: Eat, Drink— But Don't Breathe the Air!

Crowded housing conditions, smoke-filled air, bacteria-laden water, chemical pollution. London in 1850? New York in 1900? Your city in 1980? Today's large urban centers, despite major improvements in medical and health care facilities, may be hazardous to our health.

The quality of water we drink, the air we breathe, and the food we eat have been, and continue to be, critically important environmental health influences. Recent additions to this list are noise, solid waste, radiation, and toxic chemicals. These influences are part of our "physical" environment. Potentially harmful, too, are aspects of our "psychosocial" environment such as stress, crowding, and our own health habits. Their effects will be explored in subsequent chapters.

## THE WATER WE DRINK

Water quality remains the most important environmental health influence today. We take our clean water supplies for granted. Most of us have never experienced the devastating diseases that can result from contaminated water.

Water is used for drinking, personal cleanliness, and in the preparation of food. Water supplies become contaminated from organic changes — wastes — from man and animals. Normally, bacteria are filtered out as water seeps through soil. Waterborne illnesses include typhoid and paratyphoid fevers, "dysentery," cholera, and infectious "hepatitis." Microorganisms causing these diseases are found in the intestinal and urinary discharges of people carrying the diseases, including people whose symptoms are "subclinical." The phrase "toilet-to-mouth pipeline" is a colorful but not very appetizing way of describing how bacteria may be carried by water from infected individuals to our household faucets.

Today, in addition to threats to clean water through ineffective treatment of sewage and waste, man has added his own contaminants, including substances originally introduced for safety reasons. Chlorine has been cited by some people, including Nobel laureate Joshua Lederberg, a leading geneticist, as a possible cause of genetic mutations. Concerns have also been expressed about sodium fluoride, a substance added to water supplies to prevent dental decay in children. Anti-fluoridation and anti-chlorination groups are invariably found wherever health officials suggest altering so-called "pure" water supplies.

The fact is that there is no such thing as pure water. All water, no matter what the source, contains various chemicals, minerals, and bacteria. Early tests for water purity were of the "eyeball" type. It was assumed that cloudy water or water with visible particles was impure. Today's improved methods of testing water safety have made us aware of this oversimplified view. Water with visible particles may or may not be unsafe to drink. Moreover, water that is not adequate for drinking purposes may be perfectly adequate for industrial use.

Modern engineering methods for the delivery of safe water originated in ancient times. The ancient Romans drew their water supplies from distant sources through a system of 14 aqueducts totaling about 59 miles (95 km). Their system delivered over 50 million gallons (190 million litres) each day. Since each delivered water of different quality, wine was often added to the water to kill bacteria. Water arriving in Rome was stored in 12 reservoirs and distributed through mains 12 inches (about 30 cm) in diameter. Pipes were made of lead or earthenware but the Romans preferred earthenware because they already had some understanding of the dangers of lead poisoning. The general water supply was channeled into hundreds of fountains and public baths, causing most residents to obtain their own water or have it delivered by public carrier. Similar methods for transporting and distributing water were used by the ancient Greeks.

As the influence of the Greek and Roman culture spread across Europe, their methods for handling water were adopted as well. Aqueducts were built in Germany in Cologne, Bonn, Mainz, and Treves and in France at Paris, Nimes, Arles, and Lyon. Remains of aqueducts can be found today in Spain and in England.

———

Dysentery: An infectious disease of the large intestine resulting in diarrhea, blood in the stool, and other symptoms.

Hepatitis: An infectious disease caused by a virus that affects the liver. Serum hepatitis refers to transmission of the virus by hypodermic needles.

Subclinical: The presence of a disease process in the absence of obvious symptoms.

These sophisticated urban water systems collapsed in the Middle Ages. Invading civilizations and rapid urban growth led to the deterioration of ancient aqueducts and distribution mains. Cities outgrew their original supplies and began to explore new water resources. Gravity was the major source of power; conduits were built to carry the water. In 1236, King Henry III of England authorized the construction of 12 conduits to bring water to London. In the sixteenth century, pumps were used to increase the distance for water delivery to cities where gravity could no longer provide the driving force. People or horses provided power for early pumps; by the end of the eighteenth century, James Watt's steam engines powered the water pumps. The early aqueducts introduced the first large-scale supply of water for the urban public.

## SEWAGE TREATMENT

Large bodies of water can naturally purify small quantities of sewage and waste materials. A large urban population produces so much sewage that soil bacteria can no longer cope with the heavy load. As cities grow, their added volume of sewage stimulates more bacterial action. This action can deplete the oxygen and raise the temperature of streams or rivers that carry raw sewage. Bass and trout die; other fish such as carp take over. Eventually, no fish can survive. Similar changes take place with plant life. Over time, noxious gas is produced and the stream or river is unfit for recreation as well.

As the urban population increases, more complex treatment of waste materials is necessary. Generally, this involves routing organic solids into large, airless tanks called sludge digesters. Anaerobic (non-air-breathing) bacteria process this waste as a temporary measure. Effective purification requires secondary treatment involving further bacterial processing and special filtration processes. In densely populated countries where adequate processing does not occur, such as India, diseases like cholera and typhoid are common. Table 3.1 shows the historical development of water treatment processes from 2000 B.C. to the twentieth century. No major advances in technology have taken place in over 60 years.

Despite the importance of clean water, government efforts to clean up polluted waters and to prevent further pollution have not been very successful. Safety measures are often opposed by industry on the grounds that they will mean higher prices, or that they violate individual rights. Environmentalists are accused by industry of being overly cautious, particularly where there have been no recent and devastating epidemics to justify their claims. As a president of one major U.S. company declared:

> If all these nature kooks had their way, America would still be a wilderness from coast to coast. Thank God there are at least a few businessmen who care about the Gross National Product.

Table 3.1.
History of Water Treatment Processes and
Water Distribution Milestones

| 2000 B.C. | Boiling | Egypt |
|---|---|---|
| 312 B.C. | First Roman aqueduct, Aqua Appia | Rome |
| 98 A.D. | Settling reservoir and first engineering report | Rome |
| 8th Century | Distillation | |
| 1582 | First pump | London |
| 1627 | Coagulation | England |
| 1652 | First American supply work | Boston, Mass. |
| 1685 | Slow sand filtration | |
| 1761 | First steam pumping | London |
| 1800 | General use of iron pipe | England |
| 1804 | First municipal sand filter supply | Paisley, Scotland |
| 1829 | First large municipal sand filter supply | London |
| 1873 | First constant supply system | London |
| 1881 | Rapid sand filtration | |
| 1885 | Water softening | |
| 1885 | Water bacteriology | |
| 1891 | Aeration | |
| 1895 | Iron and manganese removal | |
| 1899 | Ozonation | |
| 1900 | First municipal rapid sand filter supply report | Louisville, Ky. |
| 1904 | Copper sulfate usage | |
| 1907 | Chlorine disinfection | |
| 1917 | Ultraviolet ray disinfection | |

Yet isolated examples of successful government and public cooperation to decontaminate major water supplies attest to the possibility of
success. For example, in Munich in the late 1800s Max Pettenkofer
stated that health status was related to city water and sewage systems.
Munich's deaths from typhoid dropped from 150 in 1871 to only 14 in
1875 following Pettenkofer's introduction of simple sanitary measures.
A joint cleanup by government officials and citizens of the Willamette
River in the state of Oregon in the late 1960s provides another example
of how concerted citizen action can reduce pollution.

## OTHER WATER POLLUTANTS

The purity of water in relation to bacterial infection was the major concern of early health officials. Today's water supplies face new dangers from man himself. Industrial wastes and, increasingly, wastes from nuclear power stations and oil spills pose major threats to water purity. Each day sees hundreds of millions of gallons of contaminants dumped into our water supplies: lead, detergents, sulfuric acid, hydrofluoric acid, phenols, ethers, benzenes, ammonia, pesticides, and others. These pollutants have reached such a high level that once healthy lakes and rivers no longer sustain life. As a result of the level of pollutants it contains, the Cuyahoga River running through Cleveland, Ohio, is actually inflammable!

The United States recently established an Environmental Protection Agency (EPA). The agency sets and enforces standards for the amount of chemical and bacteriological contaminants in urban water systems. Violators may be prosecuted and fined. The effects of this legislation are now beginning to have an impact on water quality. Other problems remain, however, in relation to the quality of air in the city.

## THE AIR WE BREATHE

Air, like water, used to be judged unfit on the basis of its disagreeable odor and appearance and today's judgments are not very different. The contemporary city dweller is painfully aware of burning sensations in the eyes and itching in the throat caused by air pollution. Some scientists estimate that about 25 percent of the 50-75,000 annual deaths due to respiratory diseases such as "bronchitis," "emphysema,"

—⁀—

Chronic bronchitis: An inflammation of the lining of the bronchial tubes. When the bronchi become inflamed and infected, airflow to and from the lungs becomes difficult; heavy mucus may be coughed. Bronchitis mortality rates are highest in the lower socioeconomic classes.

Emphysema: An abnormal inflating of the lungs which makes breathing difficult. It results from a loss of lung tissue. Air sacs become overly stretched to make up for lost tissue.

Asthma: An obstruction of the bronchioles which carry air from the trachea to the lungs. A reaction to internal infection or an allergic reaction to physical substances such as pollen, dust, food, or emotional stimuli. During an asthma attack a person feels as if he is choking; he cannot inhale or exhale air. Frequently one coughs up white sputum.

and "asthma" in the U.S. could be avoided if urban air pollution were reduced by 50 percent.

Pollution results when nature's natural cleansing action cannot cope with the amount of waste it must handle. It cannot cope with 66 million tons of carbon monoxide, 1 million tons of sulfur oxides, 12 million tons of nitrogen oxides, and tons of other materials such as tetraethyl lead (according to the U.S. Public Health Service, 1971).

Carbon monoxide or oxides of nitrogen interfere with cell metabolism and may place a critical strain on people with heart or lung diseases. In air with 80 ppm (parts per million) of these substances, the capacity of the circulatory system to carry oxygen is reduced by 15 percent – equivalent to a loss of a pint of blood – over an eight-hour period. Man breathes almost 31 pounds (360 cu. ft.) of air daily.

## HEALTH NOTE

### Emphysema

Emphysema in cigarette smokers in St. Louis is four times as prevalent as in cigarette smokers in Winnipeg. St. Louis is far smoggier than Winnipeg. In New York State the rate of lung cancer for men in smoggy Staten Island is 55 per 100,000; it is only 40 per 100,000 in a less smoggy area a few miles away.

In 1958 a survey in the U.S. found that the lung cancer rate in rural areas was 39 per 100,000, but more than 52 per 100,000 in cities with 50,000 or more people. These differences were found even when smoking habits and ages were taken into account.

## HEALTH NOTE

### Some Research Results

● Air pollution especially affects school-aged children. One study found that children in more urban areas in Britain had more frequent and serious middle ear and lower respiratory tract disorders than children who lived in rural areas with cleaner air.

● In San Marino, California, the performance of high school track runners was found to be poorest when there were high levels of oxides polluting the air.

● In another study it was found that British postal workers in central London who worked out of doors had more chest illnesses than did postal workers who worked indoors.

Carbon monoxide is also associated with mortality and morbidity rates. Carbon monoxide poisoning can lead to headache, loss of vision, decreased muscular coordination, nausea, and abdominal pain. Excessive amounts of sulfur oxides can lead to severe respiratory illness, particularly in older people with chronic lung disease. Hydrocarbons such as the benzopyrene molecule and some particulate substances such as asbestos also cause certain types of cancer.

Air pollution is the by-product of an affluent society. Waste emissions have increased at a more rapid rate than even the rate of population. It is estimated that while urban population will double by the year 2000, air pollution will triple if new control measures are not enforced.

In 1970 the U.S. Congress passed a Clean Air Act. This act set strict standards for air quality. For automobiles, emissions of hydrocarbons and carbon monoxide were to be reduced by 90 percent by 1975 and emission of nitrogen oxides by 90 percent by 1976. Catalytic converters in our automobiles are helping to reduce hydrocarbon and carbon monoxide emissions. But other goals of the act are not being met. Economic recession and energy shortages have led to delays in reaching the nitrogen oxide goal of the act. Unless the public renews its demands on the government to enforce the standards, it is unlikely that the ambitious goals of the Clean Air Act will ever be reached.

## SOLID WASTE

In ancient cities and some fairly modern ones as well, both organic and solid waste have been piled in open dumps, buried on land, or poured directly into large bodies of water such as lakes, rivers, or oceans. Aside from the unpleasant appearance and stench these practices create, they provide breeding grounds for disease vectors – rats, cockroaches, and flies.

Today's industrialized nations have added enormously to these concerns. The U.S. produces, annually, over 55 billion cans, 26 billion bottles and jars, 65 billion metal and plastic bottle caps, and more than .5 billion dollars worth of various types of packaging material as solid waste. In addition, about 7 million automobiles weighing almost 200 million tons are scrapped each year in the U.S.

Unplanned city growth is dangerous to our health in two ways: (1) it cuts down on the land available for waste disposal and (2) it creates more refuse. In order to protect health in the city, alternative methods to solid waste disposal must be found. These include hauling refuse to distant sites, or landfill of bodies of water. The first alternative is

---

Vector: An animal or insect that carries disease, e.g., the anopheles mosquito in the case of malaria.

extremely expensive; the second poses pollution hazards to the water itself. More recently recycling has been proposed as a solution to the solid waste problem. However, recycling programs have not been very successful to date. If we do not make major changes in the production of solid waste, for example, utilizing reusable or "biodegradable" containers, we will be drowned in an ocean of throwaway bottles and cans, empty fried chicken containers, and other "symbols" of our affluence. The state of Oregon and many others now charge sizeable deposits for soft drink bottles. Some regions have banned cans as containers. The public must demand control where governments are slow to respond.


## NOISE POLLUTION

Traffic, jackhammer drills, and supersonic jets make cities noisy. Does this noise influence our health? Yes. Excessive levels of sound can damage both physical and mental health, particularly when noise assaults our senses over a long period of time or where we have no control over it.

A brief exposure to intense noise can cause temporary loss of hearing acuity; permanent loss of hearing follows chronic exposure to high noise levels. Noise may be a factor in stress-related diseases such as peptic ulcers, high blood pressure, and emotional disturbances.

Noise is usually measured in decibels (db). The decibel scale is logarithmic; therefore a tenfold increase in sound strength is a 10-db increase. Table 3.2 gives decibel values of some common sounds. Levels as low as 50 to 55 db may interfere with sleep and cause fatigue.

The effects of excessive sound levels are elusive because, unlike bacteria, they are indirect. Recent studies in San Francisco found a relationship between the amount of measured sound on city streets and the amount of social interaction among its residents. The less sound, the more interaction. People were most dissatisfied with their living situations on streets with moderate rather than heavy levels of sound.

Noise especially influences health in the work environment. Large industrial developments and factories are usually located in or near urban areas. This means that noise may be a greater problem in cities than in rural settings. To offset these effects, businesses use devices to soften and mask noise, such as white noise – air conditioning and piped-in music. Some people find these masking devices themselves to be a source of stress. While noise and its effects are relatively obvious, certain other environmental hazards, such as radiation, are more subtle.

---

Biodegradable: Capable of being rapidly transformed into organic waste.

Table 3.2. Decibel Levels of Some Common Sounds

| sound | level (db) |
|---|---|
| Threshold of hearing | 1 |
| Normal breathing | 10 |
| Leaves rustling in breeze | 20 |
| Whispering | 30 |
| Quiet office | 40 |
| Homes | 45 |
| Quiet restaurant | 50 |
| Conversation | 60 |
| Automobile | 70 |
| Food blender | 80 |
| Niagara Falls, at base | 90 |
| Heavy automobile traffic, jet passing overhead | 100 |
| Rock band music | 100 |
| Jet taking off, machine gun at close range | 120 |

# RADIATION

In 1896 Henri Becquerel discovered "radioactivity." His work, and the work of the Curies with radium, resulted in our current concepts of nuclear energy and ionizing radiation.

We live in a "sea" of background radiation from cosmic rays and radioactive substances in the earth's crust. This background amounts to an average of 0.08 to 0.15 "rad" (a rad is the customary unit of radiation) per year.

Radioactivity: The process of giving off energy or particles by the disintegration of atomic nuclei.

Certain types of cancer, genetic defects, and stillbirths are associated with the natural background of radiation. Man-made radiation increases the incidence of health problems. William Roentgen, in 1895, produced radiation using a variation of the cathode ray tube. He called his device the X-ray. Over 90 percent of our exposure to man-made radiation comes from medical and dental uses of X-rays for diagnosis and therapy. Ironically, one of the major problems for our urban health is our sophisticated medical services and X-ray facilities.

Data from the American Heart Association and the U.S. Department of Health, Education, and Welfare indicates that during 65 years of life, each person loses approximately 64 days of life from medical and dental X-rays (see table 3.3). Prolonged and frequent radiation, often used in certain cancer treatments, can result in severe skin rashes, loss of hair, and may even produce malignancies. The head of health physics at the Oak Ridge National Laboratory in the United States believes that unnecessary medical radiation exposures today may cause between 3,500 and 36,000 deaths each year.

Table 3.3. Life Expectancy Lost or Gained
Per 65 Years Due to Radiation
and Other Factors

| | |
|---|---:|
| Fallout from all atomic weapons tests to date | -1.2 days |
| Cosmic rays, sea level | -22 days |
| Wearing luminous dial watch | -26 days |
| Cosmic rays, 5,000 feet | -33 days |
| Living over sedimentary rock | -50 days |
| Medical and dental Xrays | -64 days and more |
| Living over granitic rock | -94 days |
| Living in brick or concrete homes | -100-200 days |
| 25% overweight | -1,300 days |
| Living in the city (in contrast to rural living) | -1,800 days |
| Sedentary, in contrast to an active life | -about 1,800 days |
| Smoking, one pack per day | -3,300 days |
| Diabetes, insulin controlled | -3,600 days |
| Women, in contrast to men, will gain | +1,100 days |
| Married people will live longer than single people by | +1,800 days |

Source: Rick Carlson, The End of Medicine, New York: 1975. Data from the American Heart Association and the Department of Health, Education, and Welfare. Reprinted with permission.

Excessive levels of radiation affect future generations by changing the mutation rates of our genes. Mutations are alterations in the substances that make up the chromosomes, the carriers of the genes. These substances include DNA and RNA which when altered in one cell can carry this change on to other cells during mitosis, or cell division. The U.S. National Council on Radiation Protection indicates that there is a direct relationship between radiation dose and effect; the higher the dose, the more the effect. They state that from conception to 30 years of age a person should receive no more than ten rad of radiation.

Fallout from nuclear testing is another potential source of harmful radiation for both city and rural dwellers. Barry Commoner, a leading U.S. critic of energy policy, wrote that radiation fallout had probably caused about 5,000 defective births in the United States population up to 1963. Above ground testing of nuclear weapons was banned in 1963 by the United States, Britain, and the Soviet Union, but continues today in other countries such as France and China.

Nuclear reactors which are used to generate electric power can be another source of radiation hazard. Potential radiation leakage may occur during the mining and processing of uranium and plutonium, during power generation itself, or in the storage of long-lived radioactive wastes. These wastes must be isolated from the earth's "biosphere" for centuries. Accidental leakage from their storage and transportation could have disastrous consequences for thousands of people in nearby cities. Other dangers associated with radiation include thermal pollution from water which is used to cool nuclear reactors. A possible "accident" at one nuclear plant could release larger quantities of radioactivity than hundreds of nuclear bombs.

## TOXIC CHEMICALS

Toxic chemical substances including pesticides and excessive levels of trace elements such as lead, mercury, and zinc pose a major threat to health in the city today. These chemicals are found in food and in other

---

Mutations: Alterations in genetic structure.

DNA (Deoxyrybonucleic Acid): Part of the genetic material that controls the development of the organism. Found in the chromosomes of cells.

RNA (Ribonucleic Acid): Acid that is present in the cells along with DNA. It plays an important part in protein synthesis.

Biosphere: The part of the earth's crust, waters, and atmosphere where living organisms are found.

substances we use daily. Accidental poisonings of young children from toxic substances in dyes and paints are common.

Pesticides and related substances in our foods can pose hazards. Most mother's milk in the U.S. once contained so much DDT, a widely used pesticide, that it would have been illegal to serve under interstate commercial standards. Farmers' crops still often exceed the legal limit for residues of insecticides. Inspection is inadequate. Governments have not yet determined which levels are safe, nor have they proven that low levels of DDT are harmless. Animal studies have provided evidence that high dosages of DDT can have "carcinogenic" effects. Other animal research has shown that DDT can cause sex hormone changes and produce sterility, at least in laboratory animals.

Polychlorinated biophenyls (PCBs), another class of "chlorinated hydrocarbons," are also serious urban pollutants. They are released into the environment as vapor from storage containers, factory smoke, industrial wastes dumped into rivers and lakes, and as particulate matter from automobile tires. Other chlorinated hydrocarbons are present in low concentrations in drinking water, fruits and vegetables, the air we breathe, and in meat, fish, and eggs.

These toxic substances pose a major threat to health in the city, though certainly less than did the food preparation and handling practices 100 years ago. Still the urban dweller must rely more heavily on others to inspect and regulate the safety of his foods than does his rural counterpart. Strict enforcement of public health standards, however, can minimize the hazards of toxic chemicals.

Carcinogenic: Cancer producing.

Chlorinated Hydrocarbons: Chemical compounds that have been shown to be pollutants. DDT is the best known.

## HEALTH NOTE

### DDT And Death

A study based on human autopsies showed an association between DDT in fat tissue and cause of death. Concentrations of DDT and its derivatives were significantly higher in fat patients who died of deterioration of the brain tissue, brain hemorrhage, high blood pressure, liver damage, and various types of cancer than in those who died of infectious diseases. The history of these patients showed more use of home pesticides. Dieldrin, a pesticide which is four times more poisonous than DDT, has been implicated in a form of cirrhosis of the liver, and benzene hexachloride may contribute to liver cancer.

## SUMMING UP

Water, air, waste, and other elements of our physical environment pose problems for health in the city as do excessive levels of noise, toxic chemicals, and radiation. Yet, while the size and complexity of the city creates these hazards in the first place, the expertise and resources found in the city can also lead to their reduction and even elimination. Technologies to handle waste products and to repurify our air and water are being developed all the time. The danger is that technological advances may be outstripped by our so-called affluence.  Most industrial research is geared toward increased production; little is aimed at health protection. This balance must change, and quickly, if we are to have cities to protect.

# 4 The Residential and Social Environment: Don't Fence Me In!

> We shape our buildings and afterwards our buildings shape us.
>
> — Winston Churchill

Who are your neighbors? Could you call upon them for help if you needed it? Is your neighborhood clean and attractive? The way our cities are built strongly influences our patterns of family and social relationships, cultural values, and health practices. Physical designs can provide a breeding ground for disease-bearing rats, or lead to hazardous traffic patterns which cause accidents. They can also influence our access to emotional support from other people and thus affect our susceptibility to illness and our ability to obtain health care. The impact of our residential and social environments on health in the city is enormous.

## THE RESIDENTIAL ENVIRONMENT

Social scientists have always been interested in the influence of such factors as family relationships or patterns of social contacts — elements of the social environment — upon our health. But only recently have

> The price paid in adapting to an uncongenial environment may be difficult to estimate in money, sickness, inefficiency, and turnover, but it is too high if we can design congenial environments for the same money or less.
>
> — Robert Sommer, Personal Space: The Behavioral Basis of Design, 1969, p. 171.

they begun to recognize how these social factors are related to the physical environment, particularly the "residential environment."

"Urban ecology" examines the relationship between residential and social and health conditions. Urban ecologists take census-type data about people and their housing and find out how this information differs among areas with different rates of disease. Some recent findings:

- In the U.S., areas with crowded dwellings (more persons per room) have more hospital-treated cases of tuberculosis, chronic disabilities, suicide, infant mortality, and mental disorders.

- In Copenhagen, rates of hospital admissions for young slum children are much higher than for children living in good residential areas. Upper respiratory and gastrointestinal disorders are the most frequent cases of admission.

- Density (number of people per acre) in Copenhagen is linked with general and infant mortality, and with venereal disease, tuberculosis, mental hospital admissions, juvenile delinquency, and illegitimacy. Crowding is not linked with these problems, but is linked with suicide.

- Hospitalization for mental health problems such as psychosis, schizophrenia, and senile psychosis is usually found for areas of the city characterized by poor housing and large percentages of multiple-family dwellings.

One cannot always conclude poor health is due solely to the residential environment. High tuberculosis rates found in people who live alone as lodgers may also result from their poor housing, relocation

———

All over the world, regardless of the stage of economic and technical development, the size of the country, its political and economic systems, health services are confronted with a host of new challenges arising from "man-made" rather than "nature-made" pathogenic agents.

> – WHO Report, "Promoting Health in the Human Environment," 1974.

Residential Environment: The living unit (whether house, apartment, or hotel), the immediate surroundings, and related community services and facilities.

Sociocultural Disintegration: An index that reflects the impact of things, like social health, on the overall breakdown of a community.

and migration patterns, low income, nutritional factors, lack of social relationships, or combinations of these influences. Epidemiological mental health studies in Stirling County, Nova Scotia (Canada), in the 1950s found strong relationships between "sociocultural disintegration" and mental health. While these types of associations cannot tell us for sure what causes what, we do know that residential conditions such as housing are closely related to our health.

## Housing

Studies have found that rates for both communicable disease and accidents are as much as one-third higher in slum housing than in well-designed and maintained housing for similar families. Slum dwellers are far less likely to invite relatives and friends to their homes.

What are the direct and indirect effects of housing on health? Direct effects relate to physical structure; indirect, to things like relocation, type of housing, and density. Traditionally, health inspectors have focused on the physical side of housing: physical safety, infestation of rats and cockroaches, ventilation and heating, and other potential causes of communicable disease. These concerns are still valid. Each year dozens of city dwellers are bitten by disease-bearing rats who thrive in areas of slum housing.

A recent study of the influence of housing quality on use of health services in California found that the number of outpatient health visits dropped sharply when rats were eliminated from nearby housing developments. Such findings have led to massive rodent control programs and, at times, to relocation of residents in new low-rent housing projects.

## HEALTH NOTE

### Housing And Health In Developing Countries

In developing countries the link between the physical structure and health is clear. The World Health Organization estimated in 1968 that there were 200 million cases of elephantiasis in the world. This disease in its advanced stages causes extremely swollen legs, testicles, breasts, and other deformities. It is spread by a type of mosquito (cules fatigenes) which breeds in sewage and heavily polluted water. The most common cause is the installation of a community water supply without also installing sewers.

Proper facilities for handwashing, food preparation, laundry facilities, and proper planning to avoid traffic hazards (particularly for smaller children and older persons) are critically important to the prevention of health problems such as parasitic infections (worms, schistomiasis) and fatal accidents.

Yet, rehousing in "better" housing does not always lead to health. For example, rehoused black families, compared with white, have higher rates of tuberculosis and certain infectious and respiratory diseases, a fact that may reflect the ill effects of forced resettlement on health. Some urban health researchers have even found increases in death rates and neuroses following rehousing of slum populations to so-called "adequate" housing.

It is now clear that housing is not merely a kind of physical shelter; a residence symbolizes our identity. It has a major impact on our physical and mental health. New efforts are being made by designers to incorporate ideas from psychology and sociology into the design process. Programs in architectural and environmental psychology are providing designers with new tools and concepts for work in residential planning. Planning departments are drawing upon research in these fields, broadening their scope to include social factors as well. Just as environmental impact studies are being routinely incorporated into proposals for major economic developments – oil pipelines, for example – health impact studies must also be built into the process in years to come.

### High-Rise Strain

In cities today a major form of housing is the high-rise apartment building. Some behavioral scientists claim that high-rise living damages our health. The ideal scientific experiment needed to prove this claim would involve randomly assigning people to particular types of housing and measuring their health status regularly. One British study done in 1967 comes close to meeting this requirement. This study capitalized on a kind of "natural experiment." Groups of families of British soldiers stationed in Germany were assigned randomly to either apartments or houses. It was found that the women living in apartments paid significantly more visits to physicians than did women living in houses. The higher up they lived, the more visits they made. Their major health complaints were for nervous and respiratory conditions. There were no differences between groups in hospitalization rates. Results from these and other studies suggest that high-rise living has a major impact on psychological strain rather than on physical morbidity, especially for women.

A particular type of housing does not automatically lead to illness for everyone. Other factors, especially density and crowding, must be considered.

### Density And Crowding

By definition, urban settings contain many people, and people can be hazardous to our health. They carry bacteria and spread infection, injure us with automobiles, pollute our air and water. If it weren't for people, we might all be healthy! But people also teach us how to cope with health hazards and lend us support when we need help.  They take time to listen when stresses become distresses.

Much has been written about the ill effects of population density on health. Animal studies, particularly early work with rats, are often quoted to illustrate the disastrous effects of overcrowding. However, this early work confused the ideas of "density" and "crowding." Density and crowding do not mean the same thing. Density is a physical measure of the number of people in a certain area – say the number of people per square mile or the number of people per room. The number of people per room is found by simply adding up the number of people in a residence and dividing that number by the number of rooms in the dwelling. Four people in a one-room apartment would yield a dwelling density, then, of 0.25.

Crowding is a subjective feeling. It is related to density but is not identical with it. In his book, The Hidden Dimension (1966), the anthropologist Edward Hall pointed out that in Middle Eastern cultures or in Hong Kong a person does not feel particularly crowded even in high density conditions. But in many Western countries – England is a good example – the presence of a person even several feet away may feel oppressive. Some writers have suggested that each of us develops a kind of invisible bubble to protect our "personal space." The size and shape of this bubble is probably a result of both built-in biological devices to handle danger and learned responses. Violation of our space triggers feelings of crowding, which leads to physiological stress reactions. Prolonged stress reactions can damage our mental and physical health.

Animal studies show that even in high density conditions, as long as animals can maintain some degree of territorial control, they cope quite well. But when they lose this control, their susceptibility to health problems increases. In studies where density has been increased but territorial control has not, rats show high rates of maternal and infant mortality, reduced resistance to bacterial infection, and shorter life spans. Other animal studies have shown increases in the incidence of arteriosclerosis and neoplasms.

Do these findings apply to human beings? Probably, but only when crowding leads to disordered human relationships. Rene Dubos, the French biologist and urban health writer, states:

> The effects of crowding . . . depend on social organization and the nature of interrelationships between persons. Hong Kong and Holland are among the most crowded areas of the world, yet their populations enjoy good physical and mental health because during centuries of experience with crowding they have developed patterns of behavior that minimize social conflicts and allow persons to retain a large measure of individual freedom (emphasis added).
>
> Rene Dubos, "The Biological Basis of Urban Design," Anthropolis, p. 261.

What does Dubos mean by "patterns of behavior"? Next time you enter an elevator, observe how people behave when you say hello. Do they return your eye contact? Stand in the middle of an empty elevator and observe people's reactions as they enter. How many greet you with a smile? How about the way people act in a crowded bus or subway? Crowded situations require certain patterns of behavior to preserve privacy and safety and to reduce the potential for conflict. We are usually unaware of these rituals; we learn them as children and seldom pay much attention to them as we grow older. It is often the spontaneous behavior of little children in public places which draws these patterns to our attention. Behavior in Public Places by sociologist Erving Goffman gives an excellent description of many of the patterns of behavior to which Dubos refers.

Supplementing patterns of behavior, a well-designed residential environment can influence health in two ways. First, clean and safe housing protects us from bacteria-caused diseases. Second, housing designs that assist people to establish supportive friendships with others – while preserving their privacy – helps build feelings of well-being and a sense of community. Research indicates that these feelings may actually help us resist a whole range of stress-related physical and mental health problems. (Many of these issues are covered in chapter 5.)

## Economic Factors

Poverty is linked both to poor housing and to ill health. Poverty produces what anthropologists have called the "culture of poverty" – a whole way of life involving blocked opportunity, lack of material comfort, a shortage of resources, and a cycle of self-defeating behaviors, including alcoholism or drug abuse.

Suicide, while closely related to economic conditions, particularly reflects sudden downward shifts in economic status. During the economic depression in the 1930s, the lowest suicide rates in Britain were found among the poor while suicide rates in the formerly wealthier classes climbed to their highest levels.

The incidence of diseases such as heart disease, alcoholism, depression, and neurosis – the so-called "diseases of affluence" – are often higher for people of higher income. These problems pose special challenges to urban health because they result from the patterns of living that helped make their victims wealthy in the first place. These issues are the subject of the next chapter.

## SUMMING UP

Many studies have found relationships between the residential and social environment and illness, particularly mental illness. Poverty, unemployment, and higher population density consistently show greater prevalence of alcoholism, schizophrenia, and violent crime.

What accounts for these relationships? There are two main theories. One is that densely populated urban areas are "pathogenic." That is, they actually cause disorders by concentrating both bacteria and sources of mental stress in one geographic area. A second hypothesis says that more disease is found in the inner city because individuals and families who are likely to develop social and health problems in the first place drift to the less affluent center of the city. This "drift" idea has received support. A study in Chicago analyzed the residential location of first admission and readmission rates to a community hospital. Their maps showed a downward drift of mentally and socially disabled people toward the inner city. Health in the city both reflects and in turn influences the social as well as the physical environment.

Historically, the residential environment was inspected primarily in relation to its physical properties – water quality, sewage systems – and their impact on communicable disease. Today's residential environment still requires this type of scrutiny. But we must also inspect its social impact since today's major causes of death, the chronic diseases, reflect the social aspects of our physical environment. It is time for health inspections to include standards for social as well as physical environments.

# 5 Behavioral and Psychosocial Factors: Is it All in My Mind?

Jason and Todd live in a clean house, free of rats. The water they drink is pure. Their city's sewage system is excellent. The air is fresh. Does all this mean Jason and Todd will enjoy perfect health?

Of course not. Jason's and Todd's health depends on many inter-related factors. First there is their biological makeup – the genetic and constitutional equipment they inherited from their parents. Second, there are the environmental and residential influences discussed in earlier chapters. And, finally, there is the way the boys choose to live – their habits with regard to eating, drinking, smoking, exercising, driving, their relationship with other people, and how they cope with the stresses of everyday life. This chapter shows the influence of such behavioral risks upon our health.

Previously, the sanitation and bacterial phases of urban health paid more attention to environmental or bacterial agents than to a person's behavior. But environmental regulation of water quality and immunization practices produced exciting victories in the battle against infectious diseases.

Infectious disease prevention is a fundamental goal of health officials today. However, communicable disease is no longer the primary cause of mortality. Statistics for Vancouver, Canada, show that while in 1927 almost 40 percent of deaths were caused by infectious diseases,

---

Over 99 percent of us are born healthy and made sick as a result of personal misbehavior and environmental conditions.

John Knowles, M.D., president of the Rockefeller Foundation.

less than 5 percent were caused by infectious diseases in 1977. The prime causes of urban morbidity and mortality today are chronic diseases – heart disease, cancer – and accidents.

The scope of health service is broadening to include the practice of social and behavioral medicine. This shift is the result of changing patterns of disease, increased social consciousness on the part of twentieth-century scientists, and the development of methods in the behavioral sciences for assessing stress and modifying behavioral risks. The following section examines several of these new features and the reasons for this new focus.

## STRESS

Stress reactions, mentioned in Chapter 4 in connection with high-rise living, occur when the demands upon us exceed our capacity to cope. Demands may originate from outside – our families, jobs, economic conditions – or from internal pressures such as unrealistic standards we set for ourselves.

The physical and psychological demands of today's cities are greater than ever before but anomalies seem to exist. Large distances mean more cars and, hence, more traffic jams, yet we seem to spend little time planning and arranging for better travel. More people means more strangers and more difficult social relationships, yet we do not work at achieving better-adjusted urban associations. Cities force us to cope with these issues every day. We demand it of ourselves, yet our ability to succeed varies greatly. And when the gap between demands and our ability to cope becomes too great, stress results.

Many health problems are stress related. These "psychosomatic" disorders include peptic ulcers, high blood pressure, colitis, eczema, asthma, headaches, and others. However, increasing clinical evidence shows that stress is related to the onset and history of other diseases including tuberculosis, some heart and respiratory diseases, and some types of cancer. Stress may even lower general resistance to organic infections. Increased incidence of tuberculosis in isolated and lonely individuals supports this idea.

The popularity of the concept of stress has led to some confusion about its meaning. Some people use the word stress to mean external pressures from work, family, or urban life. Others, such as scientists like Montreal's Dr. Hans Selye, a pioneer in the field of stress, reserve the term for a consistent pattern of physiological reactions triggered by stressful external or internal events. His idea of stress differs from the concept of stress used in physics where stress refers to the applied force that tends to strain or deform a particular metal. (Selye, 1976).

Psychosomatic: Physical disorders which are often associated with emotional upset.

Selye describes three stages of stress reaction in his General Adaptation Syndrome: (1) an alarm reaction, (2) resistance, (3) exhaustion. Despite the origin or nature of stressful stimulation, a similar pattern of physiological responses follows (see Figure 5.1).

Prolonged, excessive stress can cause tissue damage. Stress stimulates the adrenal glands to secrete hormones such as adrenalin. In turn, the liver releases sugar into the bloodstream. Blood clots more rapidly, blood pressure rises, the pulse is more rapid and intense. Air passages to the lungs enlarge to admit more air. The pupils of the eyes enlarge to admit more light. Sweat breaks out, skin temperature rises or falls abruptly. At the same time, the adrenal gland releases another hormone – noradrenalin. Noradrenalin causes surface blood vessels to constrict. All this preparation for "fight or flight" is adaptive when it takes place for a short period of time. But if this stepped-up glandular activity continues over time, actual tissue damage may result.

Stress is not always harmful. It cannot and should not be avoided completely. Successful adaptation to stress may even result in an improved capacity to deal with it in the future. But where stress reactions are insufficient to cope with the situation and where, in Selye's terms, stress is experienced as "distress," physical or mental breakdown or even death can result. The specific case of heart disease offers an example of how behavioral factors, in addition to stress, can influence health (see Health Note on Type A behavior).

## HEALTH NOTE

### Type A Behavior And Coronary Heart Disease

In the mid-1960s Drs. Ray Rosenman and Meyer Friedman at Mt. Zion Hospital in San Francisco identified a pattern of behavior which predicted heart disease. They called this pattern "Type A." The pattern includes extreme

- competitiveness
- striving for achievement
- aggressiveness (sometimes strongly suppressed)
- haste, impatience, and hurried behavior
- explosive bursts of speech
- hyperalertness
- tenseness of facial muscles
- feelings of being under time pressure
- feelings of being challenged by responsibility.

Rosenman and Friedman rated more than 3,400 men as Type A or B. These men did not have heart disease. A 5½ year follow-up showed that 39-49 year old men rated Type A had an incidence of heart disease 6.5 times greater than Type B

HEALTH NOTE (Cont.)

men in the same age group.

Ironically, many Type A characteristics are those that are portrayed in popular fiction, movies, and television as the ones required for success in our hard-driving, Western, industrialized culture. Supposedly Type A traits are required for economic success and power, particularly by men.

Historically, women have had lower rates of heart disease than men. It was assumed that female sex hormones protected them against it. But recent increases in the incidence of heart disease in women are a sign that this pattern may be changing. The fact that women are taking a more active, competitive role in the marketplace may be contributing to these changes.

It is interesting to note recent comments on Type A behavior by Dr. Friedman himself. He feels that attempts to change Type A are likely to fail for two main reasons:

> First . . . because possession of Type A behavior pattern not only is a source of pride to most persons afflicted with it but it also provides them with a sense of security.

> . . . there is another reason, too, and that is that there are almost no cardiologists (heart specialists) who aren't afflicted with this same behavior pattern.

> -Dr. Meyer Friedman, "Some Thoughts on Modification of Type A Behavior," American Psychological Association, 1977.

## Work Stress

A person's work is a potential source of stress as well as satisfaction and fulfillment. It reflects his basic style of life and, in turn, affects it as well. Cities require complex stressful occupations, particularly skilled tradespeople, professionals, and managers. In contrast, rural settings traditionally involve less stressful (though no less important) agricultural and related work, including farming and ranching.

Since 1851 England and Wales have kept data about deaths in relation to occupations. Their statistics divide occupations into five broad classes ranging from Unskilled to Professional. In general, mortality decreases as the level of occupation increases. Professionals are more likely than unskilled workers to die from coronary heart disease or leukemia but less likely to die from bronchitis. Bronchitis is the leading cause of death for unskilled workers while coronary heart disease and leukemia are the least likely causes. Infant mortality rates show similar relationships; infants whose fathers are unskilled workers are more likely to die than infants with fathers in the professional or intermediate classes.

Studies also show that specific occupational groups suffer from specific health problems. For example, air traffic controllers are more likely to suffer from hypertension (high blood pressure) and peptic ulcer than comparative samples of men. Dentists have a lower life expectancy than the average white, male population. And a study of three different professions — medicine, dentistry, and law — showed higher incidence of coronary heart disease in generalists than in specialists in these fields.

As we noted in relation to housing and health, cause and effect relationships are difficult to untangle. One can never be sure whether it is occupations that cause health problems or whether the people who choose a specific occupation are prone to specific health problems. It seems clear, however, that work stress is a major factor in our health.

One way to assist workers in managing stress is the use of "relaxation" breaks. A large corporation recently instituted an experiment in which three groups of workers could choose to use their two daily 15-minute breaks either to practice a form of meditation or spend it as they normally would. For a period of 12 weeks, each group was monitored. At the end of this period, it was found that the two groups practicing meditation as a form of relaxation had experienced fewer physical symptoms, lost fewer days due to illness, improved their work performance, and increased their general level of sociability and satisfaction relative to the group that had taken its break as usual. The first two groups even reduced their blood pressures.

## Stressful Life Events

Almost 40 years ago the psychiatrist Adolf Meyer developed the "life chart." This chart was a kind of checklist that could be used to assess the impact of life events — marriage, divorce, a death in the family — on health.

In the 1960s scientists at the University of Washington developed a scale based on Meyer's life chart – the Social Readjustment Rating Scale (table 5.1). A score was assigned to each life event, expressed in Life Change Units (LCUs). What results were found?

- The higher the LCU score in the previous two-year period, the more likely it was a person would develop an illness.

- Of people with LCU scores between 150 and 199, 37 percent experienced a health change; 51 percent had a health change who scored between 200 and 299; almost 80 percent of those scoring 300+ LCU points became ill in the next two years.

- A relationship was found between increased amounts of life change and both sudden cardiac death and the timing of heart attacks.

There are a number of problems in interpreting these results. First, subjective reports about past events are often distorted as time goes by. Cardiac patients often emphasize life changes as a way of rationalizing their heart attack and as a way of denying their part in bringing it about. Also, people do not all experience the same amount of stress for the same event. Measurements that take people's unique experience of life events into account can predict future illness with greater accuracy than studies that use group averages.

The amount of stress we experience is related to the way we live. The next section examines how the way we live – our behavior and our lifestyles – influences health in the city.

## BEHAVIORAL RISKS AND LIFESTYLES

The alarm rings. You grope around and shut it off to get some extra sleep. You suddenly wake up half an hour later. You must hurry to be on time for work. You light a cigarette, gulp down a glass of juice, and jump into your car. A traffic jam. You worry that you will be late for that important appointment. This could interfere with your promotion. You light another cigarette. Finally, you arrive at the office, late. You spend the day sitting at your desk, have a few drinks at the end of the day, eat a big dinner, watch a late night TV movie, and go to bed. These habits are fairly typical for many who live in the city. But this combination of lack of exercise, poor nutrition, inadequate rest, smoking, and excessive use of alcohol all place a great strain on our physical and mental resistance to illness. They are guaranteed to increase risk for disease, particularly diseases of the heart.

The value of good health habits was recently demonstrated in a five-and-a-half-year study with 7,000 people (Belloc and Breslow, 1972). The seven habits studied were: eight hours of sleep per day, breakfast every morning, no snacks, maintaining weight within limits, no smoking,

Table 5.1. Social Readjustment Rating Scale

| RANK | LIFE EVENT | MEAN VALUE |
|---|---|---|
| 1 | Death of spouse | 100 |
| 2 | Divorce | 73 |
| 3 | Marital separation | 65 |
| 4 | Jail term | 63 |
| 5 | Death of close family member | 63 |
| 6 | Personal injury or illness | 53 |
| 7 | Mortgage | 50 |
| 8 | Fired at work | 47 |
| 9 | Marital reconciliation | 45 |
| 10 | Retirement | 45 |
| 11 | Change in health of family member | 44 |
| 12 | Pregnancy | 40 |
| 13 | Sex difficulties | 39 |
| 14 | Gain of new family member | 39 |
| 15 | Business readjustment | 39 |
| 16 | Change in financial state | 38 |
| 17 | Death of close friend | 37 |
| 18 | Change to different line of work | 36 |
| 19 | Change in number of arguments with spouse | 35 |
| 20 | Mortgage over $10,000 | 31 |
| 21 | Foreclosure of mortgage or loan | 30 |
| 22 | Change in responsibilities at work | 29 |
| 23 | Son or daughter leaving home | 29 |
| 24 | Trouble with in-laws | 29 |
| 25 | Outstanding personal achievement | 28 |
| 26 | Wife begin or stop work | 26 |
| 27 | Begin or end school | 26 |
| 28 | Change in living conditions | 25 |
| 29 | Revision of personal habits | 24 |
| 30 | Trouble with boss | 23 |
| 31 | Change in work hours or conditions | 20 |
| 32 | Change in residence | 20 |
| 33 | Change in schools | 20 |
| 34 | Change in recreation | 19 |
| 35 | Change in church activities | 19 |
| 36 | Change in social activities | 18 |
| 37 | Mortgage or loan less than $10,000 | 17 |
| 38 | Change in sleeping habits | 16 |
| 39 | Change in number of family get togethers | 15 |
| 40 | Change in eating habits | 15 |
| 41 | Vacation | 13 |
| 42 | Christmas | 12 |
| 43 | Minor violations of the law | 11 |

Reprinted with permission from T.H. Holmes and R.H. Rahe, "The Social Readjustment Rating Scale" Journal of Psychosomatic Research 11 (1967): 213-218. Copyright 1967 Pergamon Press Inc.
The scale shows the amount of stress for various life changes. The higher the point total, the greater one's chances of becoming ill.

moderate alcohol consumption, and moderate exercise. The researchers found that at age 45 those following three or less of the habits had a life expectancy of only 21.6 years while those who followed six or seven could expect to live almost 33 more. This is a difference in life expectancy of almost 12 years! And the effect is cumulative – the more health habits you follow, the greater your life expectancy and the better your health.

Do you smoke or drink? Behavioral risks of smoking, poor nutrition, lack of exercise, excess alcohol consumption, and stress are often called "lifestyle" factors. In 1974 the government of Canada published a report entitled A New Perspective on the Health of Canadians. This document emphasizes the need for governments to take behavioral risks into account in formulating health policies. A study of health policy in the state of Georgia in 1975 required experts to rate the impact of changes in each of four areas – environment, lifestyle, the health care system, and biology – on the 14 leading causes of mortality. Lifestyle was consistently rated as the area with the greatest impact for prevention of disease (see table 5.2).

A New Perspective says that since scientific knowledge is insufficient for us to be certain about behavioral risks, we must adopt the Chinese attitude of "Moi Sui" (pronounced MOO SOO) which means "to touch, to feel, to grope around" in relation to the following:

- It is better to be slim than fat.
- The excessive use of medication is to be avoided.
- It is better not to smoke cigarettes.
- Exercise and fitness are better than sedentary living and lack of fitness.
- Alcohol is a danger to health, particularly when driving a car.
- Mood-modifying drugs are a danger to health unless controlled by a physician.
- Tranquillity is better than excessive stress.
- The less polluted the air is, the healthier it is.
- The less polluted the water is, the healthier it is.

The Canadian government has embarked on a campaign called "Operation Lifestyle" to promote individual responsibility in the matters of prevention. (You can do a self-assessment of your current

---

The great inequality in the manner of living, the extreme idleness of some, and the excessive labour of others . . . the too exquisite foods of the wealthy which overeat and fill them with indigestion and, on the other hand, the unwholesome food of the poor. . . all these . . . and excesses of every kind . . . are too fatal proofs that the greater part of our ills are of our own making, and that we might have avoided them nearly all by adhering to the simple, uniform and solitary life which nature prescribed.

– Jean Jacques Rousseau, On the Origin of Inequality, 1755.

lifestyle risks using the "Lifestyle Profile" in the Appendix at the back of this book. A more elaborate assessment of risk factors using a computer-scored device called the Health Hazard Appraisal has also been developed. It is described in Appendix B.) Smoking, poor nutrition, and alcohol are its major target areas (see Health Note).

In 1976, the U.S. government published The Forward Plan for Health, fiscal years 1978-82. This report also devotes considerable attention to lifestyle factors, but does not make it part of national health policy.

## HEALTH BELIEFS

Why do people continue to smoke, overeat, and drink to excess despite evidence that shows that such behaviors are health hazards? Why does the post-heart attack victim continue to smoke heavily, work under stress, eat fatty foods, and avoid regular exercise?

The Health Belief Model shows our beliefs affect our health (see Figure 5.1). The model states that the likelihood of a person taking preventive action – like going to the dentist for a checkup – depends upon his perceived vulnerability (susceptibility) to these kinds of problems, how serious he thinks this problem might be, and the benefit he thinks will result from his visit. In addition, the person who values health highly will have better health habits than the person who does not.

Health is not valued by everyone. Health values, particularly if they are enforced through government regulations, often run counter to other values defended as "individual freedoms." Government programs of alcohol prohibition, compulsory use of automobile seat belts, and fluoridation of community water supplies have encountered massive public resistance. We are witnessing a conflict of values. Governments feel obligated to ensure the health and safety of the people and to reduce the costs of health care. Resources must be shifted to preventive health services. Individuals value their freedom to make choices about their own health behavior – even if their choices place them at risk.

⌒

Self-imposed risks, lifestyles, and the environment are the principal or important factors in each of the five major causes of death between age one and age seventy, and . . . unless the environment is changed and the self-imposed risks are reduced, the death rates will not be significantly improved.

– A New Perspective on the Health of Canadians, 1974

Table 5.2. Model for Health Policy Analysis: Disease Evaluation

| PERCENTAGE DISTRIBUTION OF TOTAL DEATHS (a) | CAUSE OF MORTALITY | PERCENTAGE (b) OF MORTALITY DUE TO EACH OF THE FOLLOWING FACTORS | | | |
| --- | --- | --- | --- | --- | --- |
| | | SYSTEM OF HEALTH CARE ORGANIZATION | LIFE-STYLE | ENVIRON-MENT | HUMAN BIOLOGY |
| 34.0 | Diseases of the heart | 12 | 54 | 9 | 28.0 |
| 14.9 | Cancer | 10 | 37 | 24 | 29.0 |
| 13.4 | Cerebrovascular disease | 7 | 50 | 22 | 21.0 |
| 4.2 | Motor vehicle accidents | 12 | 69 | 18 | 0.6 |
| 3.8 | All other accidents | 14 | 51 | 31 | 4.0 |
| 3.8 | Influenza and pneumonia | 18 | 23 | 20 | 39.0 |
| 2.7 | Diseases of the respiratory system | 13 | 40 | 24 | 24.0 |
| 2.6 | Diseases of the arteries, veins, and capillaries | 18 | 49 | 8 | 26.0 |
| 2.2 | Homicides | 0 | 60 | 37 | 3.0 |
| 1.9 | Birth injuries and other diseases peculiar to early infancy | 27 | 30 | 15 | 28.0 |
| 1.8 | Diabetes mellitus | 6 | 26 | 0 | 68.0 |
| 1.4 | Suicides | 3 | 60 | 35 | 2.0 |
| 0.8 | Congenital anomalies | 6 | 9 | 6 | 79.0 |
| | Average of percentage allocation | 11 | 43 | 19 | 27.0 |

(a) 1973.
(b) Percentages may not add up to 100 because of rounding of figures.

Source: Alan Dever, "An Epidemiological Model for Health Policy Analysis," Social Indicators Research 2 (1972): 453–466. Reprinted with permission.
COMMENT: This analysis indicates that lifestyle is the main area of health impact in 11 of the 14 areas studied.

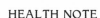

## HEALTH NOTE

### Smoking

Smoking is a learned behavior. People tend to smoke by watching others, and continue to smoke for a combination of social and biological reasons.

Smoking is clearly associated with higher death rates. Smoking more than one pack per day places a smoker in the highest risk category of all.

Recent smoking figures in Canada indicate that 37.3 percent of people 15 years of age or over report that they smoke daily. The province of Quebec led Canada in male smokers in 1975 with 50.5 percent of males reporting regular smoking while only 39.2 percent of British Columbia's males smoke. These percentages have been declining steadily since 1973. Most of the decrease is due to males. From 1965 to 1975 males showed an 11 percent decline in cigarette use while no change occurred for females.

Careful comparison studies of smoking rates for urban and rural populations are not available. However, one could speculate that since smoking is associated with social class – lower classes smoke more – then poorer, rural populations would engage in more smoking. Just how this might relate to health is not clear.

Studies of smoking habits among adolescents show that young people who smoke are strongly influenced by their social environments; those who smoke tend to associate with other smokers and to have parents who smoke, in clear contrast to nonsmokers in the same schools. Today's movements to ban smoking in public places and the increasing willingness of nonsmokers to confront smokers publicly also indicate the impact of the social environment on health behavior.

## HEALTH NOTE

### Nutrition

Nutrition is an extremely important lifestyle factor affecting health status. The history of public health offers several examples of direct relationships between nutrition and health problems. Pellagra, a dreaded disease, was found to be produced by a dietary deficiency of a vitamin called nicotinic acid, part of the vitamin B complex. Scurvy was found in 1875 to be the result of the absence of citrus fruits. Protection from the disease beri-beri is obtained from eating cured rice. This is rice that is parboiled in its husk prior to boiling. This process releases the vitamin thiamine into the kernel and makes it impossible to remove the thiamine through subsequent millings.

Nutrition has been found to be particularly important in heart disease. Increased risk of heart attack is associated with high levels of cholesterol and other fatty substances in the blood. Eating a lot of foods that are high in saturated fats, like beef, contributes to this problem. High calorie intake can also lead to extreme overweight, or obesity, another risk factor for heart disease. Excessive use of alcohol, which is high in sugar, may displace more nutritious food. A high salt intake can be related to high blood pressure, another risk factor. A recent (1977) Canadian government pamphlet on nutrition advises the following guidelines to reduce the risk of heart disease:

- Consume a nutritionally adequate diet from the four groups of Canada's Food Guide (available from your Health Department).

- Avoid becoming overweight by watching your intake of calories and increasing your exercise.

- Limit total amount of fat, sugar, alcohol, and salt.

- Increase your intake of vegetables, fruits, and whole grain cereal products.

- Include sources of polyunsaturated fatty acids (linoleic acids).

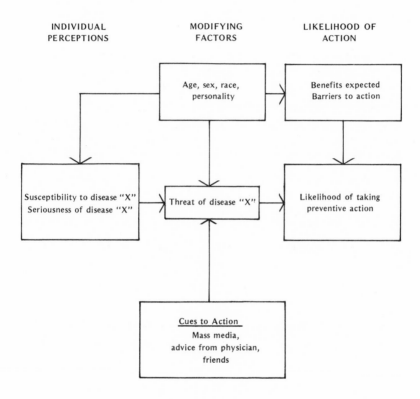

Fig. 5.1. The Health Belief Model (Simplified Form)
This model shows that preventive health action depends on our beliefs about our health and susceptibility to disease, and not simply on health knowledge alone. The fact that people have different beliefs about their health helps us explain why people resist doing what is "good" for them — like stopping smoking — even when there is clear evidence for change.

## SUMMING UP

Behavioral and psychosocial factors have a major impact on our health. As the average age of the population increases, both the incidence and prevalence of chronic disease will increase. Since the average age of city dwellers is higher than that of suburban and rural dwellers, health in the city tomorrow will depend upon our ability to decrease risks associated with chronic diseases and accidents and provide care for the elderly.

Programs of lifestyle modification which provide people with choices about patterns of smoking, drinking, eating, and managing stress are required if we are to make any progress against chronic disease and if we are to be able to pay for the increasing costs of health services.

At the same time, we cannot leave the responsibility for health entirely up to the individual. Governmental and corporate decisions also affect our health and through appropriate legislation and social action they must share the load. Examples of the need for action at this level range from issues such as fluoridation of public water supplies, nuclear energy installations and the use of pesticides to the passing of anti-smoking legislation.

---

Men are disturbed not by things but by the views they take of them.

> — Epictetus, The Enchiridion

There is nothing either good or bad that thinking makes it so.

> — Shakespeare, Hamlet

Seen on a poster:

After all the warnings I've read about the dangers of smoking, rich food, alcohol, and the need to exercise, I've come to one conclusion — give up reading!

# 6 Health Care in the City: There's Only One Thing Wrong with Hospitals— Too Many Sick People

Where do you go for health care in the city? Your first step, after discussing your symptoms with your family or friends, is to see your doctor. He or she might treat you, or refer you to a medical specialist. If your need is urgent, you might go to a hospital emergency service. For some health problems you might visit a clinic that specializes in family planning or in treating "venereal disease." You might visit your local public health unit for immunization against communicable disease. Or, you might not enter the traditional health care system at all but visit a faith healer. In a small town, your range of choices would be narrower. You would probably visit your family doctor or perhaps go to a county hospital. Only in the city would you be likely to find a broad range of diagnostic specialties and sophisticated equipment – and high costs.

Health – actually, sickness – is big business. The cost of health, including medical and dental practice, hospitals, community health centers and clinics, nursing homes and rehabilitative services, medical supplies and equipment, drugs, and dozens of other services in the U.S. amounted to over $100 billion in 1975, about 8.4 percent of the gross national product. They are expected to have reached $206 billion by 1979, about 9.1 percent of the GNP. Canada's health costs are also about nine percent of the GNP. The U.S. cost represents an increase from only $3.6 billion in 1929.

What about costs of health care in the city? New Yorkers spent an average of $855 per person on health services in 1975 for a total cost of $6.7 billion. Per capita costs in Sydney, Australia, were $863 (1974); in

---

Venereal Disease: Any of sexual contagious diseases such as syphilis and gonorrhea contracted through sexual intercourse. Usually cured by injections of penicillin.

Toronto, approximately $400 (1975). The lowest per capita costs in the U.S. are in the less urbanized Southern states.

All Western nations show a pattern of increasing costs for health care relative to other expenditures. Hospital costs are rising the fastest — over 500 percent since 1950 in the U.S. In Western cities the hospital is the center of the health care universe. Today's hospitals account for well over 90 percent of health care budgets. Yet some critics believe that hospitals no longer deserve their sacred place at the center. Ivan Illich argues that not only has the "medicalization" of our lives produced little of benefit for overall health status, it may actually be harmful. In his book Limits to Medicine (1976), Illich writes, "The medical establishment has become a major threat to health." (Illich may have a point. In spite of all our health spending, there has been no appreciable increase in life expectancy or, for many, the quality of their health. In fact, the life expectancy for American males in their middle years has actually begun to decline!)

## HEALTH PLANNING

Coordination of health services in the city is a massive task. Greater London's 16 health areas contain 36 health districts to service over 7 million people. This area alone includes 12 specialized teaching hospitals. Perhaps because of England's National Health Service, planning is more coordinated. Inclusion of health-related social services in the planning process is another benefit of their comprehensive approach (see Health Note).

## HEALTH NOTE

### Health Care In Big Cities

In 1976, the International Hospital Federation published a report entitled Health Care in Big Cities. The cities included London, New York, Toronto, Sydney, Mexico City, Bogota, Manila, and Hong Kong.

While each city's needs and services were found to be unique, four common issues emerged from the study. These issues included (1) the need to coordinate services through overall planning; (2) the fact that major health problems cannot be solved solely through the provision of hospital and medical treatment services; (3) the fact that the causes and solutions of urban health problems are not only medical, but are part of the social, political, and economic fabric of the city; and (4) the enormous cost of services.

The need for better mechanisms to plan services was recognized in the U.S. in 1974 when federal legislation created Health Systems Agencies (HSAs). The responsibilities of these agencies are:

To improve health status, increase accessibility, acceptability, continuity, and quality of health services, restrain increases in cost, and prevent unnecessary duplication of health services.

Each HSA covers a region of approximately 500,000 people. It must develop a total health plan for that region. So far only a few comprehensive health plans have been formulated and approved by the HSAs. The effectiveness of the HSA approach to health planning will depend on a great deal of cooperation among various health agencies. At this point, cooperation has not been great. Most HSAs are running into major roadblocks from hospitals and other health agencies. Rather than trying to create a new planning authority, it might have been more effective to expand the authority of existing boards of health. In fact, overall health planning was one of the fundamental reasons these boards were established in the first place!

## HEALTH CARE AND MODELS OF HEALTH

The previous chapter examined the impact of personal health beliefs on health behavior. Our collective health beliefs influence the kinds of health services our cities provide and the way these services are planned, organized, and funded.

Health services in cities reflect our Western view of man as a machine. When something goes wrong with the human machine, we expect a physician to pinpoint the trouble and repair it. Repair shops take the form of hospitals and clinics. The model further assumes that the trouble is in the machine itself. For the most part, the environment in which the machine operates is ignored. While some variations in this model take the physical and social environment into account, the repair shop model of health service is the dominant model today.

The health care system, for all its facilities and for all the numbers, training, and dedication of its health professionals, still tends to regard the human body as a biological machine which can be kept in running order by removing or replacing defective parts, or by cleaning its clogged lines.

– A New Perspective on the Health of Canadians, 1974

Specialists service each part of the machine. The more specialized the part, the greater the prestige and financial reward accorded the specialist. The smaller the machine fragment to be repaired, for example in neurosurgery, the greater the financial reward. Often the result of this specialization, though certainly not the intent, is fragmentation of the patient.

A goal of a healthy lifestyle within a healthful environment requires us to recognize that man is more than a machine whose defects require repair. Man is only one element in an ecological system consisting of other people, buildings, air, water, and foods.

## THE ECOLOGY OF HEALTH

The science of ecology is the study of reciprocal – or exchanging – relationships between organisms and their environments. These relationships hold true from the single-celled organism to an entire planet. The inventor, philosopher, and designer, Buckminster Fuller, has captured this thought vividly in his phrase "spaceship earth."

In any system, survival depends on a balance of functions at all levels of organization. If a group of cells begin to grow uncontrollably, for example as in cancer, the organism may be destroyed. The study of man's interaction with his physical and social environment is called "social ecology." In general, the study of social ecology is related to

### HEALTH NOTE

#### Hospitals In The Nineteenth Century

Hospitals in the 1800s probably caused more disease than they cured. They seldom had running water. If they did, the water was contaminated. Garbage and human waste was piled high in corridors; surgeons did not "scrub" before an operation. Many patients contracted fatal infections while in the hospital. The great Hungarian obstetrician, Ignaz Semmelweis, noted in a Vienna hospital in 1846 that high death rates from infection could be traced to the fact that students who dissected cadavers also operated on live patients without first washing their hands. The patient death rate was cut to zero when Semmelweis made hand-washing compulsory. Louis Pasteur's discovery of airborne microbes led to the introduction of antiseptic preparations into surgery. Postoperative infections were dramatically reduced. The famous surgeon, Joseph Lister, was knighted for his development of antiseptic chemicals.

epidemiology (discussed in Chapter 1) in the same way that the study of health is related to pathology.

An ecological viewpoint means that health services cannot be designed in isolation from social, political, and economic considerations. The World Health Organization at its 1974 Assembly strongly endorsed the integration of strategies to improve physical, mental, and social well-being in communities.

An ecological approach also means that we must confront our priorities. Each person does not necessarily have a right to an intensive-care unit to treat his coronary problems. Every community does not have a right to its own fully equipped hospital. Lung cancer and cirrhosis of the liver will never be prevented or reduced while governments continue to subsidize the tobacco and alcohol industries.

Ecological principles also have important implications for health practice. They mean that diagnosis must take into account not only the individual and his symptoms, but the environment(s) in which he lives. Health professionals must be involved more actively in helping to assess and change social as well as physical environments that produce disease. Prevention must become as important as cure.

Despite the fact that most governments and health professionals agree that "an ounce (gram) of prevention is worth a pound (kilogram) of cure," we still spend over 95 cents of each health dollar in the city on treatment and cure rather than on prevention. This is a serious mismanagement of priorities.

Yet some major but isolated community prevention efforts have been launched. The Stanford Heart Disease Prevention Program in Palo Alto, California (see Health Note), and the North Karelia Project in Finland are examples of two successful large-scale efforts to use massive community education and screening programs to reduce the incidence of heart disease. Unfortunately, without an overall structure to ensure their continuity, isolated prevention projects, no matter how successful, are dead-end affairs. The fact that the highly successful Stanford project no longer exists is a sad comment on current attitudes toward preventive health in the city.

Finally, an ecological viewpoint means that the center of health care shifts from the hospital to the community. New programs of homecare nursing, long-term care, and community mental health care have shown that with proper back-up resources, individuals who formerly might have been hospitalized can be maintained in their communities. A shift to community-based treatment may not only save money, it may also provide more humane treatment than hospitalization.

An example of this type of community-based approach is the system of comprehensive community health centers established in Israel by Kupat Holim Klalit (The Sick Fund of Israel's Federation of Labor) over the past twenty years. The ultimate goal of each center is to take on the responsibility for the health of every member of the community, the well and the sick. It maintains ongoing surveillance of the community's health through surveys by actual health examinations; detects immediately any increase in the incidence of infectious disease among its patients and provides the entire community with protection against it; immunizes the children of the community against measles, polio, smallpox, whooping cough, tetanus and diphtheria; provides the elementary schools in the community with health services; has an entire department devoted to mother and child care that starts at pregnancy and continues postnatally; carries on a home care program for the chronically sick and disabled who are home-bound; has its own pharmacy for filling prescriptions; has its own laboratory for blood analysis, etc.; has an independent dental clinic on the premises; has a child psychiatric unit; has a community organizer who is also a health educator and who is the liaison with all other health care agencies with which the center works — the regional hospital, the mental health center and the welfare center.

The ideal community health center will even check the water, air and food in the community regularly for contamination, going to

## HEALTH NOTE

### Stanford Heart Disease Prevention Program

One of the most effective community efforts to change lifestyles has been the Stanford Heart Disease Prevention Program. Three northern California towns were included in this project to test the effectiveness of mass media campaigns on heart disease prevention. Two communities received extensive campaigns and in one of them face-to-face counseling was used as well. The campaign consisted of 50 television spots, three hours of television programming, over 100 radio spots, several hours of radio programming, weekly newspaper columns, newspaper advertisements and stories, billboards, posters, and printed material mailed to participants. A specialized campaign was prepared for Spanish-speaking people. The third community did not receive a campaign and was used for purposes of comparison. Citizens (35-39-year-old men and women) were interviewed and examined before the campaigns and one to two years afterward. Their knowledge and behavior were assessed for dietary and smoking patterns, blood pressure, weight, and cholesterol levels.

In the comparison community, the risk of cardiovascular disease increased over a two-year period. But in the treatment communities, there was a "substantial and sustained decrease in risk." Face-to-face counseling helped make initial improvement greater, particularly in helping to reduce cigarette smoking, but the two treatment communities reached similar levels of improvement by the end of the study.

legislative lengths where necessary to eliminate it; and it will educate the community in personal hygiene and home sanitation.    The total community becomes the patient; the family becomes a basic unit of treatment by a family physician, with the complete history of every member of every family kept updated through an ongoing recording system.

## TOWARD A HOLISTIC MODEL: THE TAO OF HEALTH

An alternative to the machine-shop model of health and health care is a holistic model. It emphasizes the importance to health of diet and fitness, and the prevention of disease and the promotion of good health through the cultivation of healthy habits of living. Already many medical and health professionals are practicing within a "holistic health" model.

## SUMMING UP

Health care in the city has been traditionally centered in hospitals. Even if we could afford the continually escalating costs of sophisticated and expensive personal equipment, an emphasis on cure and treatment alone will not significantly improve health in the city.

If health care in the city is to improve, more money and resources must be shifted from treatment to community-based care and preventive services. This will require planners and politicians to adopt an ecological viewpoint and to shift from a machine-shop to a holistic model of health. Improvements in health will be made only with accompanying improvements in the quality of our social, political, economic, and educational institutions. The ancient Greeks and Romans believed that health involved a "sound mind in a sound body." A holistic model would change that phrase to "a sound mind in a sound body in a healthful city."

## HEALTH NOTE

### The Tao Of Health

The Tao (pronounced dow) refers to the branch of Chinese philosophy concerned with observation and study of nature and its Way or Tao. "Yin" refers to the dark, receptive, complex, intuitive element of nature, and is traditionally ascribed to the female; "yang" is the strong, active, rational side, traditionally ascribed to the male. These elements alternate eternally in cyclical movement to produce a whole. Traditional Chinese medicine is based on the balance of yin and yang in the body, and illness is seen as a disruption of this balance.

# 7 Health in the City Tomorrow: A Return to Hygeia, the City of Health

This book has examined present and previous influences on health in the city. Its main theme, expressed in the first chapter, is that contrary to popular belief, health in the city today is better than it was 100 years ago, particularly in relation to mortality from communicable disease. Chapter 2 outlined the history of some current health problems and described pioneering efforts at social and health reform. Chapter 3 dealt with the physical environment and health. It pointed out that while improvements in the quality of city water have reduced mortality from typhoid and cholera, air and noise pollution as well as the hazards of radiation and toxic chemicals are contributing to higher rates of morbidity and mortality from chronic respiratory diseases and certain types of cancer. Chapter 4 discussed the social and residential environments and health. Housing, crowding, poverty, and the psychological and behavioral factors mentioned in Chapter 5 are discussed in relation to three of today's major killers – heart disease, suicide, and accidents. Finally, Chapter 6 emphasized the limits to the money and manpower we can afford to spend for health in the city.

This chapter considers the future of health in the city. Can we ever achieve the ideal of Hygeia, the City of Health? In 1875 Benjamin Ward Richardson, a physician, presented his vision of an ideally healthful city. He called his book Hygeia: A City of Health. His utopian city was devoted completely to the prevention of disease and the promotion of health. The primary method used to achieve this ideal was environmental sanitation. Richardson's aim was

> . . . to show a working community in which death. . . is kept nearly as possible in its proper or natural place in the scheme of life. . . .

> – Richardson, 1875; cited in Dubos, 1965

Richardson limited his city to 100,000 persons. He provided a limit of 25 persons per acre; houses could not exceed four stories in height. The use of tobacco had disappeared; people did not use alcoholic beverages. A "principal sanitary officer" headed a small army of medical officers, registrars, sanitary inspectors, chemists, and scavenging personnel. This group of people dealt with sickness in the community. To inhibit the high infant mortality rate, which was the plague of the nineteenth century, Richardson suggested a large number of public homes where trained nurses would care for infants and small children. For the rest of the populace of Hygeia there was a system of model hospitals.

Richardson's vision had a profound impact in both England and America. Hygeian residences and Hygeian household products became extremely popular. Yet despite all this excitement, Richardson's vision was never fully realized.

Why did Hygeia fail? The reason is that major biological discoveries shifted scientific and public interest from Richardson's environmental sanitation approach to an approach based on direct medical intervention through vaccination. At the height of Richardson's popularity, scientists such as Louis Pasteur in France discovered that infections were caused by microorganisms (1864); between 1890 and 1896 vaccines for rabies, diphtheria, and typhoid were quickly developed and introduced into medical practice. By the turn of the century India was using vaccines to begin to control both cholera and bubonic plague. The hopes and dreams of Hygeia aroused by Richardson's environmental approach were forgotten. New dreams of health through "magic bullets" of vaccines took their place. It was believed that magic bullets would eventually be discovered for every disease, since all diseases were thought to be caused by bacteria. Not only would a magic bullet approach be cheaper, it would mean less change in cherished social customs and personal health habits.

We now know that neither Richardson's environmental sanitation approach nor Pasteur's magic bullet approach alone will lead to Hygeia. Despite the fact that huge sums of money are still granted each year for the search for magic bullets to cure or prevent everything from cancer to schizophrenia, more and more recognition is being given to Richardson's early emphasis on environmental sanitation. In addition we are witnessing the reemergence of an emphasis on personal responsibility for healthier lifestyles (discussed in Chapter 5). Together these three approaches – environmental, medical, and behavioral – constitute an important holistic approach. Can we now build upon Richardson's vision and current knowledge to return to the ideal of Hygeia, the City of Health?

## HEALTH AND CITY PLANNING FOR HYGEIA

Hygeia, while probably never attainable, is a worthwhile goal. However, we will need to make some basic changes in our approaches to both health and city planning. "Planning is the design of a desired future and of effective ways of bringing it about." – R.C. Ackoff (cited in Amara, 1979).

Health planning deals with the allocation of resources to reduce illness and promote health. Traditionally, health planning has been sickness planning – the building of facilities such as hospitals or clinics in which to treat the sick. Particularly in urban areas this has meant spending massive sums of money on high technology treatment. Too much of our health dollar is spent unselectively on high cost, high technology treatment resources such as hospitals and kidney dialysis units. Too little is spent on lower technology and lower cost treatment resources like neighborhood clinics and paramedical personnel. Little systematic use is made of low cost, low technology, preventive efforts to involve volunteers and citizens in the health system.

If we are ever to attain the goal of healthier cities tomorrow we need to drastically change health priorities today. We need to shift our spending from higher technology to lower technology treatment and from treatment to prevention. More responsibility for health must be placed upon citizens themselves, but with appropriate support services and incentives. Education for health must be included in schools as part of an overall life skills curriculum.

Our society must restructure various sickness benefit plans and insurance schemes, and its methods of reimbursing individuals and health professionals to reward health. This means, for example, that medical insurance plans must restructure their payment schedules. Preventive health services such as nutrition counseling must be covered. Premium discounts must be given – and in fact already are in some areas – to people whose use of alcohol is moderate and who do not smoke.

Future health planning must channel more resources into ensuring that new babies are both healthy and wanted. Prospective parents must be given the support and assistance they need to keep their babies that way. Prenatal and postnatal services – the ultimate foundation for the entire health system – require more support and knowledge from health professionals and citizens alike.

We must find alternatives to our overdependence on alcohol and drugs for stress relief. Studies show that Canadians 15 years of age and older consumed 27 percent more alcohol in 1974 than in 1966. Tranquilizers and related sleeping medications are used by almost 40 percent of the same age group, particularly by women. A 10 percent surcharge on these drugs could be used to fund research on alternative techniques to cope with stress and other topics in behavioral medicine.

And what of city planning itself? Health planning cannot be effective in isolation from overall city planning. How can we plan our cities today so that they will be healthier tomorrow? C. A. Doxiadis, a planner from Greece (also the birthplace of Hippocrates, the "father" of medicine), states:

Our present-day city is inhuman. . . .It is becoming more so with every day that passes. If it is inhuman it cannot be better for the health of mankind; it creates grave problems for man.

— C. A. Doxiadis, "The Inhuman City," Symposium on Health of Mankind, 1967

The most dehumanizing aspect of today's city is that, as a result of cars and mass transit, man has lost his freedom to move in a human scale. Population density is not the problem. In fact since 1900 the average city density in North America and Europe has dropped from 80 to less than 30 persons per acre. But lower densities combined with larger travel distances mean less direct human contact and communication.   And, as we saw in Chapter 5, less human contact means less opportunity to develop supportive social relationships which protect against stress and disease and provide access to help.

We cannot abolish cities and return to country life. We have to work with what we have. We must, therefore, design our cities to match people's basic spatial and personal needs. Doxiadis points out that the ideal space for living and traveling is 2,000 by 2,000 yards — about a ten-minute walk. Depending upon the level of density we are willing to accept, this basic "cell" can accommodate an average of about 40,000 people, and still promote healthy individual and family growth and development. Doxiadis argues that we should redesign our cities on the basis of such cells. In order to attain Hygeia we must fit the city to man's needs rather than fit man to the city's needs.

# Appendixes

# Appendix A:
# Health Statistics
# and Health Resources

## HEALTH STATISTICS

Health statistics include: "vital statistics" on important life events such as birth, marriages, and death; "demographic data" on age, sex, ethnic composition, and other characteristics of the population; and "disease data" on rates of mortality (death) and morbidity (disease). Health statistics are used to compare changes in a population's health and to compare the health of different populations at the same time. To allow such comparisons, health statistics involving the "prevalence" (number of cases in a population at a given time) or "incidence" (number of new cases in a population over a period of time) of disease are expressed as rates rather than in absolute numbers.

These statistics are used to generate hypotheses about the reasons for different rates of death and disease and can lead to prevention programs. For example, the death rate from heart disease is much higher in the U.S. than in Japan. We can compare the countries in relation to diet, smoking patterns, and other factors known to be related to heart disease incidence to see whether they differ significantly on one or more of these dimensions. If they do differ, we may have found a clue to the reason for their different rates. In fact, diets in the U.S. and Japan show marked differences; the Japanese diet includes far more fish, while diets in the U.S. emphasize beef. Experimentation could then be undertaken to follow up these kinds of hypotheses.

## HEALTH RESOURCES

Current local data on vital statistics (births, deaths, marriages):

Contact your municipal or regional Health Department.

75

National health data:

U.S. Department of Health, Education, and Welfare
Public Health Service, Health Resources Administration
5600 Fishers Lane, Rockville, Maryland 20852

National Center for Health Statistics,
U.S. Department of National Health and Welfare
Public Health Service, Health Resources Administration
Center Building, 3700 East-West Highway
Hyattsville, Maryland 20782

Canada:

Statistics Canada
Ottawa K1A 0T6

Operation Lifestyle
Information Directorate
Health and Welfare Canada
Ottawa, Ontario K1A 0K9

Britain:

Department of Health and Social Services
Alexander Fleming House
Elephant and Castle
London S.E. 1
England

International:

The United Nations Demographic Yearbook,
published biannually, is the best source
of world health, economic, and demographic data.


## OTHER INFORMATION SOURCES

### Organizations

International Hospital Federation, 162 Albert St., London, NW1 7NF,
England, Mr. Miles Hardie, Director. A forum for world information on health facilities planning and hospital care. Publishes the
journal, World Hospitals. In 1977 published the report, Health
Care in Big Cities.

World Health Organization (WHO) Headquarters, 1211 Geneva 27,
Switzerland. Publishes many journals and technical reports on
health problems and planning around the world.

Laboratory for Clinical Stress Research (WHO Psychosocial Center),
Fack, S-104 01 Stockholm, Sweden

## Journals

Environment and Behavior. Quarterly journal dealing with the impact of man-made environment on human behavior. Sage Publications, Inc., 275 South Beverly Drive, Beverly Hills, CA 90212.
(Inquiries from outside U.S. to: Sage Publications, Ltd., 28
Banner Street, London C1Y 8QE, England).

International Journal of Health Services. Quarterly journal dealing
with policy, planning, administration, and evaluation of health
services. Baywood Publishing Co., 43 Central Drive, Farming-
dale, NY 11735.

Mazingira: The World Forum for Environment and Development.
This journal's title means "environment" in Ki-Swahili, a lan-
guage spoken in East and Central Africa. It emphasizes the
global interdependence of people in the world's 150 (plus) countries today. Pergamon Press, Fairview Park, Elmsford, NY
10523.

Journal of Behavioral Medicine. Quarterly journal devoted to fur-
thering our understanding of physical health and illness through
the knowledge and techniques of behavioral science. Plenum
Publishing Corp., 227 W. 17th St., New York, NY 10011.

# Appendix B:
# Health Games

A variety of games and other materials are available to make learning about health in cities more interesting.

Lung Association Bingo (1974)
Illinois Lung Association
725 South 26th Street
P.O. Box 2576
Springfield, IL 62703

Grade: Elementary-Adult        Participants: 1-40
Time: 10 minutes-2 hours       Cost: Unknown

A packet of bingo games related to specific health problems such as cigarette smoking, ecology, and respiratory diseases.

Go to Health (1973)
Dell Books
750 3rd Ave.
New York, NY 10017

Grade: 7-Adult        Participants: 2-10
Time: 30 minutes-2 hours       Cost: $3.95 (contained in a book
                               entitled Go to Health)

Players move around a board making choices with regard to health, wealth, or security. Players must answer health-related questions correctly to proceed through life. Success in the game is based on the degree to which persons make accurate decisions affecting their health status.

Community Target: Alcohol Abuse (1975): Harry Silas, Jim Spears
Center for Health Games and Simulations
Department of Health Science and Safety
San Diego State University
San Diego, CA 92182

Grade: 9-Adult                    Participants: 3-30
Time: 4-5 hours                   Cost: $6.00

Through role playing, participants define the nature and extent of
the alcohol problem in their community and determine strategies
and programs for reducing it. In booklet form with role sheets and
instructions.

Drug Debate (1970): Karen Cohen
Academic Games Associates
430 E. 33rd St.
Baltimore, MD 21218

Grade: Jr. High-Adult             Participants: 8 pro and 8 con
Time: 2-7 hours                   Cost: $25.00

Eight drugs are debated by participants arguing from opposing points
of view. Teams attempt to compile influence points based on the
clarity of their debated position.

To Drink or Not to Drink (1972)
Games Central
55 Wheeler Street
Cambridge, MA 02138

Grade: 7-Adult                    Participants: 5-15
Time: 2-3 hours                   Cost: $26.50

A board game where players decide whether to drink alcohol or to
abstain. The consequences of drinking and its effect on lifestyle are
problems that the players face during the game.

Horse is Boss (1971): Thomas Rundquist
Thomas Rundquist
109 Virginia Park
Detroit, MI 48202

Grade: 7-Adult                    Participants: 2-4
Time: 2-3 hours                   Cost: $6.00

Simulates experiences common to chronic drug abusers involved in
illegal hustles. Participants move around a game board which
includes businesses, drugs, parties, and prostitution. Players run
risks from overdose to jail.

The Pollution Game (1971): Fredrick A. Rasmussen
Houghton-Mifflin Co.
One Beacon Street
Boston, MA 02107

Grade: 7-Adult                    Participants: 4-5
Time: 2-3 hours                   Cost: $10.41

A board game simulating the progressive pollution of our environment. Participants try to reverse the process by passing antipol-
lution measures which, if not carefully planned, result in a lethal
environment.

Ecology (1970): Bert Collins, Richard Rosen, and Margie Piret
Damon Educational Division
80 Wilson Way
Westwood, MA 02090

Grade: 7-10                       Participants: 2-4
Time: 1-3 hours                   Cost: $10.00, deluxe, $7.00, smal-
                                  ler version

Participants assume the roles of leaders of population groups. The
participant who successfully brings his/her population, technology,
and natural environment into a workable balance wins.

Smog (1970): Judith Anderson, Helen Trilling, and Richard Rosen
Damon Educational Division
80 Wilson Way
Westwood, MA 02090

Grade: 7-Adult                    Participants: 2-4
Time: 2-4 hours                   Cost: $11.00

Players assume the roles of elected officials responsible for air
quality. They confront pollution problems, making decisions that
affect financial status, popularity, growth of the town, and quality
of the air.

An "11-22" Project Review Simulation for HSA for Training (1977):
    Allan Steckler
Allan Steckler
School of Public Health
University of North Carolina
Chapel Hill, NC 27514

Grade: Adult                      Participants: 10-16
Time: 2 hours                     Cost: $2.50

The setting for this simulation is a project review committee meeting at which application of a nursing home to expand its facilities is reviewed and voted upon. Materials developed include the staff analysis of the application, proposed guidelines for project review, ten role descriptions, questions for discussion, and an evaluation questionnaire.

Mental Health (1975): Tiff Cook and Paul Ploutz
Lawhead Press
900 East State Street
Athens, OH 45701

| | |
|---|---|
| Grade: 7-Adult | Participants: 2-6 |
| Time: 1-3 hours | Cost: $8.00 |

Participants learn to deal with anxiety and stressful situations through the use of different coping techniques. The problems faced by participants simulate those encountered frequently by young people.

Physical Education Game Model (1973): Kenneth Tillman
Kenneth Tillman
Physical Education Director
Trenton State College
Trenton, NJ 08625

| | |
|---|---|
| Grade: College | Participants: Teams of 7 |
| Time: 2-5 hours | Cost: Unknown |

The objective of this simulation is to define physical education and critically analyze other definitions. Participants role play and assume different, sometimes opposite, definitions of fitness and health.

The Fit-Kit (1976): Canadian Department of National Health and Welfare (English and French versions)
Fit-Kit
Ottawa, Ontario
K1A 0S9

| | |
|---|---|
| Grade: Young adult and up | Participants: Individuals |
| Time: As required for each activity | Cost: $4.95 |

This kit is designed to help individuals measure and improve their physical fitness. Includes the Canadian Homes Fitness Test (a long-playing record which has musical cadences adjusted for different age groups); the Walk-Run Distance Calculator; the Rx for Physical Activity; the Fit-Kit Progress Chart; and a copy of the booklet Health and Fitness.

The Health Hazard Appraisal (HHA) (1979 edition). For information and forms write:

Health Hazard Appraisal
c/o Dr. John H. Milsum
Division of Health Systems
Department of Health Care and Epidemiology
University of British Columbia
Vancouver, B.C., Canada

Grade: Senior high-adult        Participants:    Individual (can do
                                group scores)
Time: 15-20 minutes             Cost: $2.00 per HHA

The HHA provides a computerized assessment of your health status based on current health risks in relation to smoking, drinking, driving, exercise, blood pressure, cholesterol, driving safety, and others. A computerized printout indicates your age in terms of your health habits relative to your actual age. (Example: Your actual age is 18 but your heavy drinking and smoking patterns put your health age at 45!) It also provides suggestions about how to improve your score.

# Annotated
# Bibliography

Amara, Roy. Strategic Planning in a Changing Corporate Environment, Long Range Planning, 1979, 12: pp. 2-16. This theoretical article, written by the President of the Institute for the Future, outlines models for long-range planning which are applicable not only to corporate life but also to health and urban planning.

Belloc, N.B. and Breslow, Lester. Relationship of Physical Health Status and Health Practices, Preventive Medicine, 1972, 1: 409-421. A very important prospective (follow-up) study which supports arguments for the positive health impact of simple health habits.

Blake, John B. Public Health in the Town of Boston, 1630-1822. Cambridge, Mass., Harvard University Press, 1959. Describes in vivid detail the epidemics and other public health problems that led to Boston's first board of health.

Calhoun, John B. Population Density and Social Pathology", Scientific American, February 1962, pp. 139-148. (Scientific American Offprint #444.) One of the classic studies of the physical and social effects of overcrowding.

Carlson, Rick. The End of Medicine. New York: John Wiley, 1975. A provocative analysis of the changes taking place within the medical and health fields today; includes a forward by Ivan Illich.

Cities: Their Origin, Growth, and Human Impact. Readings in Scientific American. San Francisco: W.H. Freeman and Co., 1973. Articles about cities that have appeared in Scientific American. Excellent graphics and well written.

Davies, William H. The Complete Poems of W.H. Davies. London: Johnathan Cape Ltd., 1935. This volume of his collected poems includes many of his most beautiful love poems written during the 1920s and '30s.

Davis, Kingsley. The Urbanization of the Human Population. In Cities, Scientific American, Inc.: New York: Alfred Knopf, 1969. One of a collection of articles dealing with various aspects of city life. Unfortunately none of the papers deals directly with health in the city.

Doxiadis, C.A. (ed.). Anthropolis: City for Human Development. New York: Norton Publishing Co., 1975. Some of the leading thinkers in the field including Rene Dubos, Erik Erikson, Margaret Mead, C.H. Waddington, and others discuss ways to make the city of tomorrow a more human place in which to live. A bit heavy, but worth the effort.

Doxiadis, C.A. The Inhuman City. In Health of Mankind, Gordon Wolstenholme and Maeve O'Connor (eds.). London: J. & A. Churchill Ltd., 1967.

Dubos, Rene. The Biological Basis of Urban Design. In Anthropolis (already cited), pp. 253-263. The brilliant biologist examines how individual biology must be taken into account in designing cities and how density and human interaction must be seen within a biological context.

Duhl, Leonard. The Urban Condition: People and Policy in the Metropolis. New York: Basic Books, 1963. One of the first books to focus people's attention on the impact of urban life on people.

Friedman, Meyer. Some Thoughts on Modification of Type A Behavior. Paper presented to the American Psychological Association, San Francisco, 1977. A brief, informal paper which provides some behind-the-scenes insights into the personal as well as scientific aspects of research on the relationships between Type A behavior and coronary heart disease.

Gans, Herbert J. Planning – and City Planning – for Mental Health. In Taming Megalopolis. Vol. II. H. Wentworth Eldredge (ed.). Garden City, N.Y.: Anchor Books, 1967. An example of an effort by an urban sociologist to raise public awareness of the impact of city life on mental health and the need for planners to pay more attention to such issues.

Goffman, Erving. Behavior in Public Places. Garden City, N.Y.: Doubleday, Anchor Books, 1963. A fascinating study of the rituals people display in meeting and interacting together in public settings by one of today's keenest public observers.

Holmes, T. & Rahe, R.H. A Social Re-adjustment Rating Scale, Journal of Psychosomatic Research, 1976, 11: 213-218. For the measurement-minded, an account of the development of this widely-used research tool.

Illich, Ivan. Medical Nemesis: The Expropriation of Health. London: Marion Boyars Publishers Ltd., 1976. Professor Illich is a scholar whose sizzling writing indicts the health system. Although overstated and dramatic at times, the book is a must for advanced students in this field.

Insel, Paul M., and Moos, Rudolf H. Health and the Social Environment: Issues in Social Ecology. Lexington, Mass.: D.C. Heath & Co., 1974. Outlines basic issues and research in the field of social ecology, the study of social environments on human behavior.

Insel, Paul M., and Roth, Walton T. Health in a Changing Society. Palo Alto, Calif.: Mayfield Publishing Co., 1976. This comprehensive health textbook is both fascinating and readable. Its coverage of social and psychological factors is excellent.

Levi, Lennart and Anderson, Lars. Psychosocial Stress: Population, Environment and Quality of Life. New York: Spectrum Books, 1975. These Swedish authors are among the few to cover the impact of psychosocial factors on health and, more broadly, the quality of life. It's a good example of how epidemiological data can be used for planning health services.

Longmate, Norman. Alive and Well: Medicine and Public Health, 1830 to the Present Day. Hammondsworth, Middlesex, England: Penguin Books, 1970. A brief and extremely well-illustrated introduction to the history of public health; excellent reference material.

Macaulay, David. City: A Story of Roman Planning and Construction. Boston: Houghton Mifflin Co., 1974. Very readable, well-illustrated book showing step-by-step city planning methods practiced in early Roman times; it offers valuable lessons for planners today.

Meyer, Evelyn E. and Sainsbury, Peter (eds.). Promoting Health in the Human Environment. Geneva: World Health Organization, 1975. A special World Health review position paper which emphasizes the impact of both the physical and the social environments on world health.

Purdom, P. Walton (ed.). Environmental Health. New York: Academic Press, 1971. One of the most clearly written and comprehensive textbooks on environmental health. It deals with social as well as physical environments.

Read, Brian. Healthy Cities: A Study of Urban Hygiene. Glasgow and London: Blackie, 1970. Provides a clear outline of how traditional health problems of the environment – air, water, and waste – have been handled in urban settings.

Richardson, Benjamin Ward. Hygeia: The City of Health (1875). Cited in Rene Dubos, Man Adapting. New Haven: Yale University Press, 1965. A nineteenth century utopian vision of the ideally healthy city – Hygeia. It shows clearly the strong influence of the Sanitary Revolution in public health during the Victorian era.

Selye, Hans. The Stress of Life. McGraw-Hill: New York, 1976. The second edition of Selye's classic book outlining his General Adaptation Syndrome and related theories of stress as nonspecific responses.

Sommer, Robert. Personal Space: The Behavioral Basis of Design. Englewood Cliffs, N.J.: Prentice-Hall Inc., 1969. This little book influenced the development of the field of environmental psychology. It carefully summarized research and observations dealing with the effects of designed environments on human behavior. It has been widely read by behavioral scientists and designers alike.

Weiss, Jay M. "Psychological Factors in Stress and Disease," Scientific American, June 1972, pp. 104-113. Describes how scientists study the effects of psychological factors on disease in the animal laboratory and how these results might be applied to human beings. Clearly written and illustrated.

World Health Organization. The First Ten Years of the World Health Organization. Geneva: Palais des Nations, 1958, p. 459.

# Index

Alcohol consumption, 13-14
    and stress relief, 71
Anthropolis, 43
Antibodies, 13-14
Aqueducts, 14-15, 26
Architectural psychology, 42
Asthma, 29

Bacteria, 13
Becquerel, Henri, 33
Behavioral medicine, 47-48
Benzopyrene, 29
Bible, 14
Bills of Mortality, 21
Bio-degradable, 32
Biosphere, 35
Biostatistics, 21
Broad Street Pump, 20
Bronchitis, 29

Canadian Health Policy, 54
    Operation Lifestyle, 54
Cancer, 29
Carcinogens, 36
Cassel, John, 3
Causes of death, 1
    by age, 1
    urban vs. rural, 1-2
Central Board of Health, 22
Chadwick, Edwin, 21, 23
Chemicals, antiseptic, 64
Chemicals, toxic, 36

Chicago community hospital
    admissions, 45
Chlorinated hydrocarbons, 36
Cholera, xiii
    definition, 19
    epidemic, 19
Cholesterol, xvi
Churchill, Winston, 39
Cities, growth of, 2
Clean Air Act, 31
Commoner, Barry, 35
Converters, catalytic, 31
Coronary Heart Disease, 3
Crowding, 40. See Density, 42-43
Crude mortality rates, 9
    and causes of death, 9
    definition, 6
    Table 1.1, 10
Curie, Marie and Henri, 33

Davies, William Henry
    quotation from Love's Rival, 1
Davis, Kingsley, 2
DDT, 36
Decibels, 33
Demography, xvi
Density, 40
    vs. crowding, 6
    in cities, 71-72
De Sanitate Tuenda, 15
Diets in Middle Ages, 17-18
Disraeli, Benjamin, 11

DNA, 35
Doxiadis, C.A., 71-72
Drug use in Canada, 71
    stress relief, 71
Dubos, Rene, 43
Dysentery, 26

Ecological viewpoint, 13-14
Ecology, 64
    and health services, 65
Egyptians, ancient, 14
Elephantiasis, 41
Emphysema, 29, 30
Environmental Protection
        Agency, 29
Environmental psychology, 42
Epictetus, 60
Epidemic, 19
    in England, 15
    yellow fever in U.S., 23
Epidemiology, xvi
    definition, 5

Farr, William, 20
Fitness, 13-14
Fluoridation, 26
Forward Plan for Health, 49
Fuller, Buckminster, 64

Galen, 16
Gans, Herbert, xv
General Adaptation Syndrome, 49
Goffman, Erving, 44
Greece, 71
Greeks, ancient, 15

Hall, Edward, 43
Harvey, Sir William, 17
Health, xvi
    beliefs,
        49, 55, 59, 63
    Old English Derivation, 3
    utopian views of, 70
Health boards, 23
Health care costs, 24, 61-63
Health insurance, 71
Health maintenance organi-
        zations, 24

Health planning, 62
    in big cities, 62
    in England, 62
    and services to newborns, 71
Health Systems Agencies, 63
Health of Towns Report, 21
Henry III, 27
Hepatitis, 26
High-rise strain, 42
Hippocrates, 15, 71
Holistic health, 65
Hospitals
    in 19th century, 64
Housing, 41
    and accidents, 41
    and communicable disease, 40
    and disease protection, 44
    and health in developing
        countries, 41
    and supportive friendships, 44
    and use of health services, 41
Hydrocarbons, 36
Hygeia, 69-70

Illich, Ivan, 63
Incas, early, 14
Incidence rate, 5
Income and disease, 44
India, 70
Industrial revolution, 2
Infant mortality rates, 6
    in various countries, 6
Inoculation, 13
    smallpox, 15
Inspectors, health, 15

Knowles, John, 47

Laws, early public health, 16
    in England, 16
    in Germany, 16
    in Milan, 16
Leprosariums, 15
Leprosy, 14
    historical, 14
Life chart, 51
Life expectancy, 6-9
Lifestyles and health, 52
    need to change, xv
Lister, Joseph, 63

Magic Bullets, 70
Malaria, 15
Medical Officer of Health, 22
Meyer, Adolf, 51
Miasma, 13, 15
Micro-organisms, 70
Middle Ages, 16
Minoans, ancient, 14
Monasteries, 16
Morbidity rates, 9-11
Mortality rates, 6-7
Mutations, 35

National Health Service, 63
National Health Survey (U.S.), 11
North Karelia Project, 65
Nuclear testing bans, 35
Nutrition, 14, 58

Occupational mortality, 49, 51
Oxides, nitrogen, 29
    sulfur, 29

Pasteur, Louis, 64, 70
Personal space, 43
Pesticides, 36
Pettenkofer, Max, 28
Plagues, 17
Planning, city, xvi, 71
Planning, health, xvi, 65, 71
Plato, 5
Poisoning, carbon monoxide, 27
Pollution, air, 29-30
    noise, 32-33
    water, 25-29
Poor Laws, 21
Population, 14
    shifts since 1800, 4
    in sixteenth century Euro-
        pean cities, 2
    urban vs. rural, 3
    in year 2000, 3
Poverty and health, 44
    and suicide, 44
Prevalence rate, 6
Psychosomatic disorders, 48
Public Health Act, 23

Rad, 33
Radiation, 33-35
    x-ray, 34
    deaths from, 34-35
    days of life lost from, 34
Radioactivity, 33
Relaxation, 51
Renaissance, 16-17
Residential environment, 86
Residential relocation, 41
Revolution, industrial, xiii
    and life expectancy, xv
Richardson, Benjamin Ward, 143
Risk, behavioral factors, 47, 51
RNA, 35
Roentgen, William, 34
Rosenman, Ray, 50
Rousseau, Jean Jacques, 52

Sanitary Act, 23
Sanitary movement, 16
Sanitation, 13, 16, 18
Selye, Hans, 48
Semmelweis, Ignaz, 64
Sewage, 18
    systems in Crete, 1000 B.C., 14
    treatment, 56
Shakespeare, William, 60
Shattuck, Lemuel, 23
Smallpox, 19
    in U.S., 23
Smith, Stephen, 23
Smith, T. Southwood, 21
Smoking, 14, 57
Snow, John, 20
Social ecology, 42
Social Readjustment Rating
    Scale, 51, 53
Sociocultural disintegration, 40
Sommer, Robert, 39
Stanford Heart Disease Pre-
    vention Project, 65, 66
Steam engine, 27
Stirling County, Nova Scotia, 40
Stress, 13, 48-49
Subclinical,
    definition, 26
Suicide rates, 44

Tao, 67
Tranquilizers, 71
Tuberculosis, 40
    and housing, 41
    and social isolation, 48
Type A behavior and heart
        disease, 50
Typhoid, xiii
    epidemics, 19
Typhoid Fever, 20
Tyroler, Herman, 9

Urban ecology, 40
Urban vs. rural, death rates, xvi
    life in 1850s, 17
Urbanization, xiii, 2-3
    See also Population

Vaccines, 70
Vancouver, 47
Vector, 31
Venereal disease, 61
Vesalius, 17
Vienna, 63
Vital statistics, 20

Waste, solid, 31-32
    treatment, 13
Water, pumps, 18
    quality, 25
Watt, James, 27
Working conditions, 19
World Health Organization, 39

# About the
# Author

MALCOLM S. WEINSTEIN, Ph.D., is Director of Health Planning for the Vancouver Health Department.